English for Nurses

G.N. Prabhakara M.D.
Associate Dean
Shri Dharmasthala Manjunatheswara
College of Medical Sciences and Hospital
Manjushree Nagar, Sattur
Dharwad, Karnataka-580 009

and

Malathi Prabhakara M.A.
Formerly Senior Scientist, CFTRI
Mysore-9570013

PEEPEE
PUBLISHERS AND DISTRIBUTORS (P) LTD.

English for Nurses

Published by
Pawaninder P. Vij

Peepee Publishers and Distributors (P) Ltd.
Head Office: 160, Shakti Vihar, Pitam Pura
Delhi-110 034 (India)

Corporate Office: 7/31, Ansari Road, Daryaganj
New Delhi-110002 (India)

Ph: 41512412, 23246245, 9811156083

e-mail: peepee160@yahoo.co.in

e-mail: peepee160@rediffmail.com

g-mail: peepee160@gmail.com

www.peepeepub.com

First Edition: **2006**
Reprint: **2020**

ISBN: 978-81-8886-773-8

Preface

English an International Language also called Global Language is spoken by 630 million people across the world.

"Speaking Skill" through good Phonetics, Loud reading, Usage of correct grammar and Fluency with confidence are the need for the nurse in her profession.

Reading, Writing and Communicating in English which is the medium of the study in Nursing Profession are mandatory for an effective learning and for inter-professional interactions.

In this venture, an effort is made for presentation of Grammar, Composition, Phonetics, Comprehension and Vocabulary through usage of Professional Language (nursing profession).

This **ENGLISH FOR NURSES** is meant for nurses as per their curriculum according to Indian Nursing Council, during the placement in first year of their career.

We thank Dr. K.R. Pravin Chandra Associate Professor in Community Medicine for his help in proof-reading.

We acknowledge the effort of Mr. Pawaninder P. Vij, Director, M/s Peepee Publishers and Distributors (P) Ltd., New Delhi and his dedicated staff who gave a superb model, shape and design to our modest work which has come out as **English For Nurses.**

G.N. Prabhakara

Malathi Prabhakara

Contents

Chapter 1

Grammar

Grammar is a way a language puts across words to form long units of meaning.

1.1. LETTER, WORD, SENTENCE

There are 26 **alphabets** in English. Among them, A, E, I, O and U are Vowels. Remaining are Consonants.

When alphabets are joined and used: and give some meaning, we call them as **words.**

e. g., book, table, go, at.

We speak by using **sentences.** Sentences are group of words which give full meaning.

e. g., Mary is a good girl.
We examine a patient.
Bed making is first lesson.

Types of sentences are:

1. **Assertive sentence:** Here we make statements.
   e. g., Pooja has surgery posting.
   Matron takes a class.
   Our batch has 100 percent results.
   Show compassion for patients.
2. **Interrogative sentence:** Here we ask questions:
   e. g., Which is your native place?
   Did you complete your field posting?
   When is your internal assessment test?
   Do you want to become O.T. Nurse?
3. **Imperative sentence:** Here we command:
   e. g., Be silent.
   Show mercy on poor patients.
   You must pass in first attempt.

Take care when you are assisting surgery on HIV positive case.

4. **Exclamatory sentence:** Here we show feelings:

   e. g., What a city !
   How hot this place is !
   Oh! What a rain !!
   Such a powerful man next to *Bheema*!

1.2. SUBJECT, PREDICATE

Subject is the part which names the person or a thing we speak about. In other words we name a person or a thing.

e. g., **She** ate *Idli.*
Rama killed *Ravana.*
Cat drinks milk.
Rat flea transmits disease.

Here, She, Rama, and Rat flea are subjects.

Predicate is the part which tells something about the subject. In other words we say something about a person or a thing. In the above examples the predicates are:

Ate *idli.*
Killed *Ravana.*
Drinks milk.
Transmits disease.

Table 1.1: Subject and predicate

Subject (*names a person or a thing*)	*Predicate* (*tells something about the subject*)
She	Ate *idli*
Rama	Killed *Ravana*
Cat	Drinks milk
Rat flea	Transmits disease

First part of sentence which names a person or a thing is subject. Second part of sentence tells something about the subject and hence is a predicate.

1.3. PHRASE, CLAUSE

Group of words which do not make complete sense is called **Phrase.**

e. g., The moon shines **in the sky.**
Nurse gives **soap water enema.**
Syringes are boiled **for 20 minutes.**
Demonstrate to me how to **elicit reflex**.

Here, the phrases are:
In the sky.
Soap water enema.
For 20 minutes.
To elicit reflex.

Group of words in a sentence that contains a subject and a predicate form **Clause.**

e. g., Nurse has a ring **which is made of American gold.**

We cannot go out **while it is raining.**

Here, the Clauses are:
Which is made of American gold.
While it is raining.

1.4. PARTS OF SPEECH

Depending upon the role or part in a sentence and depending on their use, we have eight kinds of words. They are:

1. Noun
2. Adjective
3. Pronoun
4. Verb
5. Adverb
6. Preposition
7. Conjunction
8. Interjection

1.4.1. Noun

Definitions

Noun is the name of a person, place or a thing.

e. g., Rosy is a girl.
Dharwad is a calm city.
Tea poi is made of glass.

Kinds

There are four types of noun. They are **Proper noun, Common noun**, **Collective noun** and **Abstract noun.**

When name refers to a particular person, place or a thing it is called **proper noun.**

e.g., *Harsha.*
Mysore city.
Sim's speculum.

When noun refers to a name given in common class to a person, a place or a thing. It is called **common noun.**

e. g., Boy (can be other than *Harsha).*
City.
Instrument.

When noun refers to collective group containing number of persons, places or things it is called **collective noun.**

e. g., A herd of cattle.
A group of nurses.
A set of instruments.
A committee of nursing examiners.

When noun refers to the quality of describing a person, a place or a thing it is called an **abstract noun.**

e. g., A beautiful nurse.
Kind hearted Tutor.
Whole hearted Ward Nurse.
Super white cloth.

Table 1.2: Kinds of noun

Proper noun	*Common noun*	*Collective noun*	*Abstract noun*
Harrison	Pupil	Crowd	Truth
Rita	Ship	Class	Honesty
Delhi	Year	Fleet	Wisdom
Kolkota	Ward	Committee	Innocence
India	Voice	Jury	Brave

Genders

In case of Noun, we have four genders. They are Masculine, Feminine, Common and Neuter genders.

Examples:

Table 1.3: Kinds of genders

Masculine	*Feminine*	*Common*	*Neuter*
Boy	Girl	Baby	Bag
King	Cow	Cattle	Chair
Prince	Daughter	Calf	Pen

Methods or ways of forming feminine gender:

a. Using different words.

Boy	Girl
Brother	Sister
Bull	Cow
Earl	Countess
Horse	Mare
Man	Woman
Sir	Madam
Son	Daughter

b. By adding a syllable.

Count	Countess
Poet	Poetess
Hero	Heroine
Testator	Testatrix
Sultan	Sultana
Master	Mistress

c. By placing a word, before or after.

Landlord	Land lady
Peacock	Peahen
Washerman	Washer woman
Mother-in-law	Father-in-law
Step-mother	Step-father

Number:

In case of Noun, we have two numbers called Singular and Plural. **Singular** denotes one person or thing. **Plural** denotes more than one person or thing.

Examples:

Singular	*Plural*	*Remarks*
Pen	Pens	By adding 's'
Cow	Cows	
Branch	Branches	By adding 'es'
Box	Boxes	
Negro	Negroes	
Mango	Mangoes	

Contd.

Contd.

Story City	Stories Cities	'y' removal and adding 'ies'
Half Leaf	Halves Leaves	'f' removal and adding 'ves'
Scarf Dwarf	Scarves/Scarfs Dwarves/Dwarfs	Takes 's' or 'ves' for plural
Proof Kerchief Safe	Proofs Kerchiefs Safes	'f' or 'fe' takes s for plural
Foot Goose Tooth	Feet Geese Teeth	Changing the inside vowel
Child Ox	Children Oxen	By adding 'en'
Sheep Pair Dozen Hundred Series Species Aircraft	Sheep Pair Dozen Hundred Series Species Aircraft	Some nouns are same in singular and plural
— — —	Spectacles Tongs Scissors	Two parts forming a kind od pair hence nouns are always plural

Case:

In case of Noun, we have three cases which are **Nominative case**, **Objective case** and **Possessive case.**

When a noun is used as subject of a verb it is called **Nominative case.**

e. g., Bhaskar built a house (answer is got for who built the house?)

Vikram Singh shot the pig (answer is got for who shot the pig?)

When a noun is used as an object of a verb it is called **Objective case**.

e. g., Bhaskar built what ? A house (answer is got for question what?)

Vikram shot what ? A pig (answer is got for question what?)

When a noun shows ownership or origin etc., it is **Possessive case.**

e. g., Nurse's quarters.
Parvathi's dance.
Jesus' name.
Women's college.

1.4.2. Adjective

Definition

An Adjective is a word which qualifies a noun indicating
Quality
Kind
Quantity
Number
of a person, a place or a thing.

e. g., Our Nursing Tutor is a **brilliant** speaker.
The two-year-old child is **clever.**
Matron gave me **four** Moosambi fruits.
I don't have **time** for picnic.
You can operate in **that** O.T.

Here, brilliant, clever, four, time and that are adjective.

Kinds

When adjective shows the quality of a noun it is called **adjective of quality.**

e. g., Our Nursing College has a **large** hospital.
The postman in Cuttack is an **honest** man.
That criminal has not changed and is a **foolish** man.
The sky is **blue.**

When adjective shows the quantity it is called **adjective of quantity.**

e. g., Serve me **some** sambar.
Please drink a **little** water.
Your idea has **no** meaning.

When adjective shows the number it is called adjective of number.

e. g.,
The child suffering from a syndrome has **7** fingers.
My friend was the **first** to get PhD in Nursing
Senior tutor taught us **many** things.

Degrees of Comparison

Simple form of adjective in the degree of comparison is **Positive Degree**. It is not comparison at all and hence is simple one.

e. g., Sweet
Tall
Great
Fat

When two things are compared the adjective is **Comparative degree.**

e. g., Sweeter
Taller
Greater
Fatter

Table 1.4: Formation of comparative degree

Positive degree	*Comparative degree*	*Remarks*
Sweet Tall Great	Sweeter Taller Greater	By adding 'er'
Fine Able Pure	Finer Abler Purer	By adding 'r' when word ends with 'e'
Hot Fat	Hotter Fatter	Consonant is doubled and 'er' is added
Beautiful Proper	More beautiful More proper	By adding 'more'
Good Many Bad	Better More Worse	Not formed from positive degree and are irregular

When more than 2 things are compared the adjective is **superlative degree**.

e. g., Sweetest
Tallest
Greatest
Fattest

Table 1.5: Formation of superlative degree

Positive degree	*Superlative degree*	*Remarks*
Sweet Tall Great	Sweetest Tallest Greatest	By adding 'est'

Contd.

Contd.

Fine Able Pure	Finest Ablest Purest	When ends with 'e' add 'st'
Hot Fat	Hottest Fattest	Consonant is doubled and 'est' is added
Beautiful Proper	Most beautiful Most proper	By adding 'most'
Good Many Bad	Best Most Worst	Not formed from positive and are irregular

Interchange of degrees of comparison:
When there is no comparison it is positive degree.
e.g., This sister is a clever girl.
When you compare two it is comparative degree:
e. g., This sister is cleverer than that sister.
When you compare more it is superlative degree.
e.g., This sister is the cleverest girl in this nursing college.

Usage of adjective as noun and vice versa

Table 1.6: Usage of adjective as noun and vice versa

Adjective as noun	*Noun as adjective*
Rich people (plural noun)	Mexican Cowboy
Poor people (plural noun)	Circus girl
Our future (singular noun)	Computer game
Lover of beauty (singular noun)	
Indians (as noun)	
Criminals (as noun)	
Solids (as noun)	
In black and white (as phrase)	
In short (phrase)	

Correct use of adjectives

1. Little, A little and The little:

Little	*A little*	*The little*
Not much, practically nil **e.g**., There is little hope of recovery in this patient	Some but not that much **e.g.,** A little knowledge is dangerous	Available in small quantity **e.g.,** The little money received was quite useful

2. Few, A few and The few

Few	*A few*	*The few*
Not much, practically nil **e.g.**, Few people achieve perfection	Small number, not that much **e.g.,** I have a few relatives in Canada	Available in small number **e.g.,** Give the few spare clothes to him

3. Each and Every

Each	*Every*
Weak word Used for two Refers to individual of the group Used when we have limited number **e.g.**, Each bench has the capacity of 10	Strong word Used for many Refers to whole group Used when we have unlimited number **e.g.,** Leap year is once in every 4th year

4. First and Foremost

First	*Foremost*
First in the list First in the order **e.g.,** Jawaharlal Nehru was the first P.M. of India	It is prominent It is a leading item **e.g.,** Sir C V Raman was the foremost scientist of his century

5. Less and Lesser

Less	*Lesser*
Small sized e.g., I have less confidence in him	Not great at all e.g., Drowning is lesser of the two other evils

6. Some and Any

Some	*Any*
To express quantity **e.g.,** Go and buy some pickle	Used after 'if' in affirmative sentence Used in negative sentence e.g., If you need any help come to me. Do not buy any bangles

7. Other words:
   Elder and older—used only for persons
   Older and oldest—used for both living and nonliving

Nearest—nearness in space
Next—refers to position
Farther—refers to distance
Further—additional
Later and latest—refers to time
Latter and last—refers to an order
Many—It is numerous
Many a—Singular word but used as plural which refers to experience
A great many—Means a large number
Outermost—Far away from centre
Uttermost—remote
Utmost—extreme.

Article

Definition:

Since they demonstrate person, place or a thing they are called **demonstrative articles**.

They are **A**, **An** and **The.**

Kinds

'A' and 'An' are **Indefinite articles** because they are not definite.

'The' is **Definite article** because it is not indefinite.

Table 1.7: Kinds of articles

A	*An*	*The*
Indefinite Used before singular	Indefinite Used before singular Used before vowels a,e,i,o,u Used before word which sound vowel e.g., Hour (our) Honest (onest) Heir (eir) Not before 'h' if word do not sound vowel as in (horse), (hole)	Definite Used before singular or plural Used for a particular thing

How to use Articles

Table 1.8: Usage of articles

Article	*Usage*	*Remarks*
A	A boy A girl A house A year	Used before consonants
	A foot A word A cord	Used as original measure
	A boy and a girl	Used to repeat
An	An army An eye An inkpad An orange An umbrella	Used before a,e,i,o and u
	An (h)onourable An (h)onest An (h)eir An (h)our	When word sounds like vowel
The	The nurse The instrument The patient	When we speak of a particular item or person
	The rose (roses) The cow (cows)	When singular gives the meaning of many
	The West Indies The Cauvery	Used before proper names
	The Bible The Ramayana	Used before mythological texts
	The great Ravana The immortal Gandhiji	When 'noun' with adjective clause
	The nurse and the staff	To compare

No 'articles' are used under the following conditions:

No articles with abstract nouns:

e.g., Pearl is precious.
Sugar is bad.

No articles with proper nouns:

e.g., Tagore is a great poet.
Delhi is a capital.

No articles with material nouns:

e.g., Steel.
Concrete.
Gold.

1.4.3. Pronoun

Definition

This is a word used instead of a noun.
(**note**- it- is- for- a- noun)

Kinds

Personal pronoun = They stand for persons.

e.g., I, We,
You
He, She,
They

Forms of personal pronouns:

I person	*II person*	*III person*
I My Our	Thou Thy You	He Her His She They

Table 1.9: Forms of personal pronouns

Person	*Singular*			*Plural*		
	Nominative case	*Possessive case*	*Objective case*	*Nominative case*	*Possessive case*	*Objective case*
I	I	My Mine	Me	We	Our Ours	Us
II	Thou You	Thy Thine Your	Thee You	Ye You	Yours truly, Yours	You
III	He She It	His Her Hers Its	Him Her It	They	Their Theirs	Them

Impersonal pronoun = They stand for things

e.g., It,
They

Reflexive pronoun = When 'self' is added to personal pronoun

e.g., Myself
Yourself
Herself

Himself
Themselves

Demonstrative Pronoun = They point out objects

e.g., This
That
These
Those

Indefinite Pronoun = When they refer to general thing

e.g., Everyone's mouth
Few escaped
Some are great
One cannot
None believe

Distributive Pronoun = Distributes to tell one at a time

e.g., Each of the nurses
Either of these procedures
Neither is true

Relative Pronoun = It relates to noun

e.g., Meet the nurse who got the rank
Found the ring which was lost

Interrogative Pronoun = It questions:

e.g., Who are you ?
Which is the case ?
What is the matter ?

1.4.4. Verb

Definition

The verb tells or asserts something about a person, a place or a thing:

e.g., Ran
Rose
Claimed
Is
Have
Gave
Likes

The verb may have more than one word:

e.g., Was giving
Is learnt
Has been singing

Kinds

Transitive verb: When action passes over from subject to object:

e.g., Singh kicks the ball (action of kicking passes over to the ball).

Intransitive verb: When action is not passed over from subject to object:

e.g., Uma cries badly (crying is not passed over to subject).

Predication

We predicate the **act** or **action** or **verb** as complete or incomplete as far as predication is concerned.

e.g., of complete predication of verb (makes full sense)

e.g., woman sleeps
girl sings

e.g., of incomplete predication of verb (makes partial sense)

e.g., woman seems sleepy
girl seems singing

Active and Passive Voice

When 'a person does something' or 'something is done to the person' we use the word **active voice** and **passive voice** respectively.

e.g., Rai helps Pai (Rai does something). Hence active voice.

Pai is helped by Rai (something is done to Pai). Hence passive voice.

Changing Active to Passive Voice

James killed a rat.	A rat was killed by James.
Fisherman caught a big fish.	A big fish was caught by fisherman.
Kuvempu wrote a poem.	A poem was written by Kuvempu.
Child broke the mirror.	The mirror was broken by the child.
He bought an NSC.	An NSC was bought by him.

Changing Passive to Active Voice

Accidents are caused by rash driving.	Rash driving causes accidents.
Warrior was given a reward by Government.	The government gave a reward to the warrior.
By whom was this complaint sent?	Who sent this complaint?
I was given a book by Niranjan.	Niranjan gave me a book.

Mood

Mood is the manner in which an action (verb) is denoted. This can be a command, a question or a statement.

e.g., Don't go.
How are you?
He sings well.

Kinds of mood:

Indicative mood: (Statement or question)

e.g., Students are taught grammar.
Did you find that girl ?

Imperative mood: (Command or prayer)

e.g., Go to sleep!
Oh! God! Protect me from Devil.
Make me rich.

Subjunctive mood: (Desire or wishes)

e.g., Emerald stone is good for you.
God bless you!

Tense

Tense says the exact time of an action (verb).

e.g., I am shouting.
I shouted.
I will shout.

Kinds of Tenses:

Present Tense—Verb refers to present time.

e.g., She loves.
He starts.

Past Tense—Verb refers to past time.

e.g., She loved.
He started.

Future Tense—Verb refers to future time.

e.g., She will love.
He will start.

Uses:

Present Tense

Present simple	*Present continuous*	*Present perfect*	*Present perfect continuous*
I drink coffee	I am drinking	I just drank coffee	I have been drinking
You play	You are playing	You have played	You have been playing

Past Tense

Simple past	*Past continuous*	*Past perfect*	*Past perfect continuous*
I received letters	I was receiving letters	I had received letters	I had been receiving letters
He died	He was dying	He had died	He had been dying

Future Tense

Simple future	*Future continuous*	*Future perfect*	*Future perfect continuous*
I shall return	I shall be returning	I shall have returned	I shall have been returning

Verb used in different person and in different number:

First person	*Second person*	*Third person*
I sing (singular)	You sing (singular)	He sings (singular)
We sing (plural)	You sing (plural)	They sing (plural)

The infinitive verb: It is a base for the verb to signify features of a verb.

e.g.:

To make	We desire to make money.
To respect	Our duty is to respect teachers.
To operate	Doctor is there to operate on him.
To sing	Cuckoo bird loves to sing.

The Participle:

It is a verb which **acts** both **as verb** and **as an adjective.**

e.g., Hearing the bell, the boy ran to school.

The Gerund:

When we add 'ing' to use either as a verb or as a noun.

e.g., Teach me swimming.
Seeing is believing.

Irregular Verbs: They are of three types.

Same word is used in present tense basic form, past tense and in past participle:

Set	Set	Set
Cut	Cut	Cut
Hit	Hit	Hit

Same word is used in past tense and in past participle:

Bleed	Bled	Bled
Catch	Caught	Caught
Feed	Fed	Fed

All three forms are different in basic form, past tense and in past participle:

Bite	Bit	Bitten
Fall	Fell	Fallen
See	Saw	Seen

Auxiliaries

Words that help verbs to form different tense, different voice, questions and negatives:

Be (He is working)
Have (He has worked)
Do (He doesn't work)

Modals

Words used before verbs to express permission, possibility, certainty and necessity:

Can	(I can do it)
Could	(I could do it)
May	(I may do it)
Might	(I might do it)
Will	(I will do it)
Would	(I would do it)
Shall	(I shall do it)
Should	(I should do it)
Must	(I must do it)

Strong Verbs

A verb which forms its past tense by a change in the main vowel of the present tense and without the addition of any ending is called **a strong verb.**

Present	*Past*	*Past participle*
Sit	Sat	Sat
Give	Gave	Given
Bind	Bound	Bound
Hold	Held	Held

Weak Verbs

A verb which forms its past tense by adding ed, d or t to the present tense, either with or without a change in the main vowel sound, is called **a weak verb.**

Present	*Past*	*Past participle*
Feel	Felt	Felt
Post	Posted	Posted
Lead	Led	Led
Pay	Paid	Paid

A few examples of strong and weak verbs:

Strong verbs	*Weak verbs*
Bear	Hate
Fall	Deal
Swear	Bleed
Write	Bend
Hold	Catch
Spit	Hurt
Win	Tell

Verb Conjugation

By combination of parts of other verbs we make voice, mood, tense and number. It is called **conjugation.**

Example of complete conjugation of the word '**come**'.

Verb—Come

Tense—Present Tense

Simple present tense	*Present continuous tense*	*Present perfect tense*	*Present perfect continuous tense*
I come	I am coming	I have come	I have been coming
We come	We are coming	We have come	We have been coming
You come	You are coming	You have come	You have been coming
He comes	He is coming	He has come	He has been coming
She comes	She is coming	She has come	She has been coming
It comes	It is coming	It has come	It has been coming
They come	They are coming	They have come	They have been coming

Verb—Come

Tense—Past Tense

Simple past tense	*Past continuous tense*	*Past perfect tense*	*Past perfect continuous tense*
I came	I was coming	I had come	I had been coming
We came	We were coming	We had come	We had been coming
You came	You were coming	You had come	You had been coming
He came	He was coming	He had come	He had been coming

Contd.

Contd.

She came	She was coming	She had come	She had been coming
It came	It was coming	It had come	It had been coming
They came	They were coming	They had come	They had been coming

Verb—Come

Tense—Future Tense

Simple future tense	*Future continuous tense*	*Future perfect tense*	*Future perfect continuous tense*
I shall (will) come	I shall (will) be coming	I will have come	I will have been coming
We shall (will) come	We shall (will) be coming	We will have come	We will have been coming
You shall (will) come	You shall (will) be coming	You will have come	You will have been coming
He will (shall) come	He will be coming	He will have come	He will have been coming
She will (shall) come	She will be coming	She will have come	She will have been coming
It will (shall) come	It will be coming	It will have come	It will have been coming
They will (shall) come	They will be coming	They will have come	They will have been coming

1.4.5 Adverb

Definition

An **adverb** is a word which modifies another adverb, or a verb or an adjective.

e.g., This bunch of grapes is *very* sour (modify adjective).
Nurse reads *slowly* (modifies verb).
He reads *quite* clearly (modifies adverb).

Kinds

Adverb of time (answers 'when?')
I shall go there *tomorrow*.
Let us start *now*.

Adverb of frequency (answers 'how often?')
Tutor took the class *twice*.
Sister *always* helps the patient.

Adverb of place (answers 'where?')
She lives *here.*
Please come *in.*
Doctor looked *up.*

Adverb of manner (answers 'how?')
Nurse manages *skilfully.*
The English for nurses is *well* written.

Adverb of quantity (answers 'how much?')
The doctor was *partly* correct.
Ward boy was *too* careless.

Adverb of affirmation
Certainly, the B.Sc., nursing is tough.
The ward nurse *surely* is mistaken with patient.

Adverb of reason
Therefore, go to bed
Hence, you are unfit.

Interrogative adverb
Where is the patient? (place)
When are you having examination? (time)
Why are you depressed? (reason)
How do you study? (manner)
How many students are there in I B.Sc., Nursing? (number)
How cold is Kashmir? (degree)

Formation

Clever Quickquickly Beautiful	cleverly beautifully	by adding 'ly'
Ready Happy	readily happily	Change 'y', 'v' by 'ly'
Single Double	singly doubly	word ending 'le' change 'e' to 'y'
Thereby Herewith Wherein		compounded with preposition

Contd...

Contd...

By the by Now and then Off and on Over and above To and fro	two adverbs with conjunction

1.4.6. Preposition

Definition

A **Preposition** is the word placed before a noun or pronoun.

e.g., I am fond *of* sweets.

Is there any elephant *in* the field?

Kinds

There are three kinds: Simple preposition, Compound preposition and Phrase preposition.

Simple preposition	*Compound preposition*	*Phrase preposition*
By	Above	According to
At	Across	Along with
For	Along	Because of
Of	About	For the sake of
On	Among	In case of
Out	Around	In favour of
To	Before	In order to
Up	Below	In spite of
With	Between	With regard to
Till	Inside	
	Within	

Relation by Preposition

Place:	To stand *before* the door To stay *within* the house
Time:	To wait *till* 5th August To give *within* a month
Agency:	To send the letter *by* courier To cut the fruit *with* knife
Manner:	To work *with* devotion To fight *with* courage

Contd.

Contd.

Purpose:	Taking medicine *for* infection To suffer *from* skin infection
Possession:	Mexican *with* red hat Vajranna is a man *of* principle
Measure:	Site is sold *by* the meter It is 7 O'clock *by* my watch

Special Prepositions

'Than', 'But' and 'A' are special prepositions. Their usage is illustrated.

e.g., Don't accept less *than* one rupee.
What can she do *but* die?
To meet once *a* month.

Words that are always followed by particular prepositions:

Famous **for**
Subsists **on**
Fond **of**
Appraised **of**
Divided **into**
Wish **for**
Acceptable **to**
Liable **to**
Confined **to**
Match **for**
Adapted **to**
Ignorant **of**
Derived **from**
Famous **for**
Profited **by**

Impossible **to**
Indebted **to**
Contemporary **of**
Remarkable **for**
Associated **with**
Prevented **from**
Acquainted **with**
Suited **to**
Different **from**
Insured **to**

Contd.

Contd.

Addicted **to**
Susceptible **to**
Originated **in**
Judged **by**
Hints **at**
Cure **for**
Due **to**

Words that take "for" as preposition:

- Affection for
- Ambition for
- Anxiety for
- Apology for
- Appetite for
- Aptitude for
- Blame for
- Candidate for
- Capacity for
- Compassion for
- Compensation for
- Contempt for
- Craving for
- Desire for
- Esteem for
- Fitness for
- Fondness for
- Guarantee for
- Leisure for
- Liking for
- Match for
- Motive for
- Need for
- Opportunity for
- Partiality for
- Passion for
- Pity for
- Predilection for
- Pretext for
- Relish for
- Remorse for
- Reputation for
- Surety for

Common words with specific prepositions

With	*Of*	*To*	*From*	*In*
Alliance with	Assurance of	Alternative to	Inference from	Absorbed in
Bargain with	Charge of	Access to	Descent from	Accomplished in
Comparison with	Doubt of	Antidote to	Escape from	Accurate in
Conformity with	Experience of	Approach to	Exemption from	Backward in
Acquaintance with	Failure of	Attachment to	Abstinence from	Correct in
Enmity with	Proof of	Attention to	Cessation from	Defective in
Intercourse with	Result of	Concession to		Deficient in
Intimacy with	Want of	Dislike to		Experienced in
Relation with		Encouragement to		Enveloped in
		Enmity to		Fertile in
		Exception to		Honest in
		Incentive to		Implicated in
		Indifference to		Interest in
		Invitation to		Involved in
		Key to		Proficient in
		Likeness to		Versed in
		Limit to		
		Menace to		
		Obedience to		
		Objection to		
		Obstruction to		
		Opposition to		
		Preface to		
		Reference to		
		Resemblance to		
		Sequel to		
		Submission to		
		Succession to		
		Supplement to		
		Temptation to		
		Traitor to		

Related words take different prepositions:

Affection *for*	Affectionate *to*
Capable *of*	Capacity *for*
Confidence *in*	Confident *of*
According *to*	Accordance *with*
Desire *for*	Desirous *of*
Equal *to*	Equally *with*
Except *for*	Exception *to*
Fond *of*	Fondness *for*

Contd...

Contd...

Liking *for*	Dislike *to*
Negligent *in*	Neglectful *of*
Partial *to*	Partiality *for*
Prepared *for*	Preparatory *to*
Qualified *for*	Disqualified *from*
Result *of*	Resulted *from*
Respect *for*	Respectful *to*
Subsequent *to*	Consequent *upon*
Want *of*	Wanting *in*
Trust *in*	Distrust *of*

Correct use of preposition

Beside=by the side of *(house is besides river)*
Besides=in addition to *(besides speaker also an actor)*

Since = from a point of time in the past *(she is absent since 15 days)*
For = referred to a period of time *(he is appointed for 3 years)*

Between = referred to 2 persons or 2 things *(choose between 2 photos)*
Among = referred to more than 2 persons or 2 things *(a custom among Hindus)*

By = referred to doer of action *(the tiger was shot by Ranger)*
With = referred to instrument of action *(shot with rifle)*

In = refer is to a place *(he lives in Himachal Pradesh)*
At = referred to small place *(meet me at the club)*

On = more general point of time *(grand party on 17th)*
In = a period of time *(brought in the morning)*
At = exact point of time *(be there at 4 PM)*
By = show latest time of action *(leave by 6 AM)*

In = being inside *(he is in the bed)*
Into = movement to inside *(he came into room)*

On = things at rest *(he sat on easy chair)*
Upon = about things in motion *(she jumped upon her horse)*

In = at the end of a period

(space shuttle reached the moon in 3 days)

Within = before the end of period

(loan repayment within one year)

1.4.7. Conjunction

Definition

The **conjunction** is a word which joins two words or two sentences.

e.g., He and She
One or Two
Man proposes and God disposes.
The man may be poor but is not dishonest.

Kinds

Simple conjunction:
They are simple like — 'and', 'are', 'but' etc.

Correlative conjunction:
They are used in pairs.
e.g., Either .... or
Neither ....nor
Both .... and
Though ..... yet
Whether ...... or
Not only ...... but also

Compound conjunction:
They are compound expressions.
e.g., Even if
So that
Provided that
As though
Inasmuch as
As well as
As soon as
As if
In order to
On condition that

Classes of Conjunction

Two kinds:

1. Coordinating conjunction.
2. Subordinating conjunction.

Coordinating conjunction: Conjunction joining two statements of equal rank.

e.g., Husband is president and the wife is secretary.

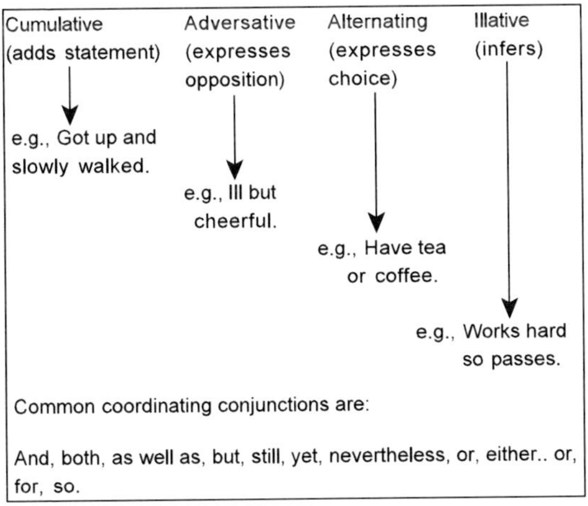

Fig. 1.1: Types of coordinating conjunctions

Subordinating conjunction:

Conjunction joining one clause to another.

e.g., When
Where
While
Before
Unless
That
Though
Till
If
Because
After
Than

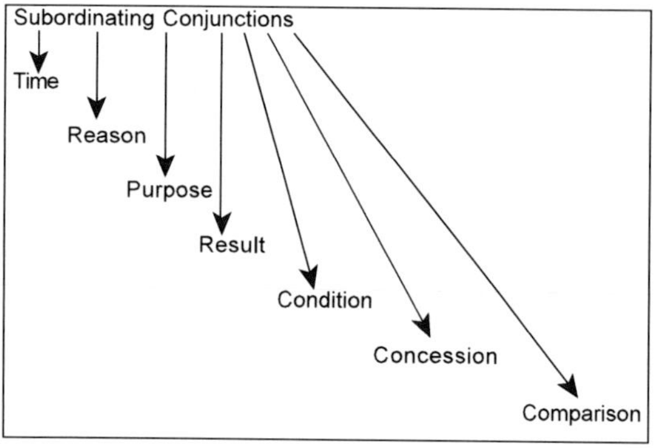

Fig. 1.2: Types of subordinating conjunctions

Examples of subordinating conjunctions connecting clauses:

Adverb clause of Time:

e.g., See me *before* you go.
Don't forget *till* death.
Serve *as soon as* it is ready.

Adverb clause of Reason:

e.g., I should go *for* I have work.
Promoted *because* he was efficient.
I will do it *since* you desire it.

Adverb clause of Purpose:

e.g., Work hard *that* you may succeed.
Have defence *lest* enemy will attack.
Play game *in order that* health improves.

Adverb clause of Result:

e.g., He was so weak *that* he could hardly stand.
She walked *so much that* she got tired.

Adverb clause of Condition:

e.g., Go to U. S. A. *if* you get scholarship.
No help *unless* you tell the truth.
It looks *as if* it might rain.

Adverb clause of Concession:

e.g., He works hard *though* he is weak.
She uses costly dresses *although* she is poor.
Book is a book *although* nothing is there.

Adverb clause of Comparison:

e.g., He is *cleverer than* I.
I like him *better than* her.
Bheema was *stronger than* Duryodhana.

Common Conjunctions

Since = From that time	*(I have not seen cinema since 40 years)*
Or = Alternate	*(Your pen or my pen)*
If = Suppose	*(If he comes I will see him)*
That = Demonstrates	*(Not that I love Caesar less, but that I love Rome more)*
Than = Compares	*(I see her often than seeing him)*
Lest = Negative purpose	*(He escaped lest he should be killed)*
While = During that time	*(While there is a will there is a way)*
Only = Except	*(Day is hot, only rather dry)*
Except = Unless	*(Except accompanied by men no other women are allowed)*
Without = Unless	*(I go without you)*

Because = Closest/causal conjunction
For = Weakest conjunction
Since = Between 'because' and 'for'

Common Correlative Conjunction

Either .... or
Either you or he will have to go.
Neither .... nor
Neither he nor she could have done this.
Not only .... but also
Not only looted but also set fire.
Not ...... but
This thief was not Akbar, but was Kalam.

Though .... yet

Though he has injury yet wants to play.

Whether .... or

Whether he comes or not, I will travel.

Both .... and

He is both scholarly and cultured.

As .... so

As you sow, so you reap.

So .... as

Patient is not so bad as you think.

So ...... that

The work is so much that one person alone can't do it.

Such ..... that

I have such regards for him that I will do anything to please him.

Such ...... as

I gave him such help as I could.

No sooner ... than

No sooner had she received the telegram than she fainted.

Scarcely .... when

Scarcely had I reached Railway Station when train steamed out.

1.4.8. Interjection

Definition

The interjection expresses sudden feeling or an emotion. **(Joy, Grief, Surprise, Approval)**

e.g., Ah !
Oh !
Hash !
Hello !

Compound expressions are also common: such as:

God heavens !!
Good Gracious !!
For shame !!
Ah me !!

Remedial study of the chapter:

1. Grammar is the way a language puts across words to form long units of meaning.
2. There are 26 alphabets which include 5 vowels *a, e, i, o, u.*
3. When alphabets are joined they form words.
4. A group of words which give full meaning is a sentence.
5. Subject is the part which names a person or a thing.
6. Predicate is the part which tells something about the subject.
7. Group of words which do not make complete sense is phrase.
8. Group of words in a sentence that contains subject and predicate form clause.
9. Depending upon the work or part in a sentence and depending on their use we have eight kinds of words.

   They are called Parts of Speech.
   - *Noun*
   - *Adjective*
   - *Pronoun*
   - *Verb*
   - *Adverb*
   - *Preposition*
   - *Conjunction*
   - *Interjection*
10. In parts of speech, we use some common words, to work for the given part of speech. They are:

The	Till	Up	Well
What	While	When	Yet
Round	Since	So	Some
Still	Such	That	No
No	Once	One	Only
Over	Right	Like	Little
More	Much	Near	Needs
Neither	Next	Except	For
Less	Any	As	Before
Better	Both	But	Down
Either	Enough	Even	Above
About	All	After	Else

11. It is the function or use that determines to which parts of speech a word belongs.

Chapter 2 Composition

The word composition literally denotes the act or method of putting the words together. This demonstrates the constitution of sentences in the language.

The composition analyses, transforms and synthesises words, phrases and sentences.

The composition also tells us the sequence of tenses and nature of speech we make, and puts them in proper depiction.

2.1. ANALYSIS

Detailed study of words and sentences in a language by studying their content, structure and pattern is called language analysis.

Nature, content, clauses and further transformation of sentences are studied.

2.1.1. Words, Sentences

Words

When letters are joined and give some meaning, we term them as "words". To make a sound or a word we need letters. But words are joined to get a meaning in conversation or writing.

When we say "He" it gives meaning and hence is a word. Suppose we write 'LLAT' it does not mean anything. The reason is that letters are not joined to give a definite meaning. The same four letters if arranged and written like 'TALL' it gives meaning and hence can be called a word.

Book, Pen, Table, Slate etc., are words.

In case of letter 'A' and 'I' they are single letters but are used to produce sound.

A BOOK, I GO are treated as words with use of single letter A and I.

All required letters should be near to each other to form a word. If we write **BO OK**, it cannot be a word. Instead **BOOK** is word.

Sentences

The Simple Sentence:

Sentence is a set with many words to give complete meaning. It contains subject and a predicate.

e.g., Rama killed Ravana.
Srihari shouts.

Rama and Srihari are subjects. 'Killed Ravana' and 'shouts' are predicates.

So, a simple sentence has only one subject and one predicate each.

e.g.,	The sky	is blue
	The cow	gives milk
	The annual sports	will be held tomorrow

The Compound Sentence:

A sentence which consists of two or more main clauses is called a compound sentence.

e.g., Krishna went to the station *and* boarded the Chennai train.
You can go by plane *or* by train.
Bharat went to Chennai, got his visa *and* came back.

Here, coordinating conjunction 'and' and 'or' are used.

The Complex Sentence

A sentence which consists of one main clause and one or more subordinate clauses is called a complex sentence.

e.g., You should do as I did.
When we went there we found that he had gone.

'You should do', 'we found' are main clauses.
'As I did', 'when we went there' 'that he had gone' are subordinate clauses.

The Compound-Complex Sentence

A sentence containing two or more main clauses and at least one subordinate clause, it is "*Double sentence*" or Compound-Complex sentence.

e.g., While the man played the harmonium, the boys sang and the girls danced.
I knew that he was ill, but I did not know that he suffered from leukaemia.

'Boys sang', 'girls danced' are coordinate main clauses.

'While the man played the harmonium' is subordinate clause,

'I knew', 'I did not know' are coordinate main clauses,

'That he was ill', 'that he suffered from leukaemia' are two subordinate clauses.

2.1.2. Phrases

Phrases are incomplete sentences.

There are three important phrases which student should observe and understand.

They are:

Adjective phrase
Adverb phrase
Noun phrase.

2.1.2.1. Adjective Phrase

It is a group of words that does the work of an adjective.

Adjective Phrase	*Adjective*
A purse without any money	Empty purse
The National Flag of India	The Indian Flag

2.1.2.2 Adverb Phrase

It is a group of words that does the work of an adverb.

Adverb Phrase	*Adverb*
Danced in a beautiful style	Beautifully
(He lives) in Turkey abroad	Abroad

2.1.2.3 Noun Phrase

It is a group of words that does the work of a noun.

Noun Phrase	*Noun*
Enjoy eating sweet	Sweet
Win the Nobel Prize	Nobel prize

Note the following illustrations to understand Phrases made suitable to Adjective Phrase, Adverb Phrase and Noun Phrase:

Adjective Phrase	*Adverb Phrase*	*Noun Phrase*
Birds **of the same feather** flock together.	Do not survey **at random.**	I don't want **to visit the Zoo.**
He lost a diamond **of great value.**	Nurse passed **in the examination.**	Professor hates **playing cards.**
Padma is a woman **of great prudence.**	Rita does her homework **in haste.**	My getting a first rank surprised **my wife.**
Draw a picture **of your nursing college.**	He has driven **in a reckless manner.**	Pretend **to know everything about first aid.**
The road leading **to the township is very muddy.**	Florence Nightingale treated her patients **with compassion.**	Child enjoys **reading comics.**

2.1.3. Clauses

Clause is a group of words which has a subject and a predicate of its own, makes complete sense and forms part of a larger sentence.

There are three kinds of clauses.They are:

Adverb Clause

Adjective Clause

Noun Clause

2.1.3.1. *Adverb Clause*

A group of word which join together to form part of a sentence and has a subject and a predicate of its own is a clause. When this clause does the work of an adverb, it is called an Adverb Clause.

e.g., Saint did *sandhyavandan* at **sunset.**
She is not as clever **as you are.**

2.1.3.2 Adjective Clause

When a clause does the job of an adjective it is called Adjective Clause.

e.g., I know the town **where the nurse lives.**
Any nurse **who comes late** will be punished.

2.1.3.3. Noun Clause

When a clause does the job of a noun it is called Noun Clause.

e.g., This is just **what I wanted.**
I wonder **what the nurse wants.**

Note following illustrations tabulated to understand Adverb clause, Adjective clause and Noun clause:

Adverb Clause	*Adjective Clause*	*Noun Clause*
He cannot see **unless he wears spectacles.**	I found the stetho-scope **that I had lost.**	I do not know **who he is.**
Do **as you please.**	No nurse **who is honest** shall suffer in any way	Please show me **how ECG machine works.**
Make hay **while the sun shines.**	The temple **which Dean is referring to** is 400 years old.	Have you heard **that the nurse is going to Paris?**
He sings exactly **as Mohammed Rafi does.**	Rama went away by plane **which departed at 6.00 AM.**	It is certain **that Pooja will get a rank.**
People do not go out **if it floods.**	Where is the diamond ring **which I purchased from "Kari & Sons"?**	**That he is a terrorist is** a well-known news.

2.1.4. Sentence

Group of words which makes complete sense is called a sentence. There are three different kinds of usage of sentence, namely, Simple sentence, Compound sentence and Complex sentence.

Sentence	*Simple sentence*	*Compound sentence*	*Complex sentence*
Criteria	Has one subject Has one predicate	Has two or more main clauses	Has a main clause Has one or more subordinate clause
Examples	I am bold. The nurse is beautiful.	She studied hard, but she could not succeed. We are guided by reason and the animal by instinct.	The college, in which I study, is very large. Whatever you do, do well

2.1.4.1. Simple Sentence

Simple sentence has one subject and one predicate.

e.g., Birds flock together.
Fire burns.
The president visited our college.
The secretary of SDM went to see the president.

2.1.4.2 Compound Sentence

Compound sentence is made of two or more main clauses.

e.g., I jump, I walk, I leap and I sing for joy.
(Note four coordinate sentences)
The night is dark and I am far from home.

2.1.4.3 Complex Sentence

Complex sentence consists of one main clause and one or more subordinate clauses.

e.g., I promised him that he would be promoted.
When the rain stopped, we set out for the next town, where we had planned to stay the night.

2.2. TRANSFORMATION

In a language we should have variety of expressions both in speaking and in writing. When we convert a sentence and mention it in different forms, the process is called as "Transformation".

This is similar to what we have seen earlier that a phrase can be changed to a sentence and a sentence to a phrase without changing their meaning.

So, transformation means changing a sentence from its one form to another without altering its meaning or its sense.

Main areas of transformation in language are:

1. Removing "too" in a sentence.
2. Changing the degree of comparison.
3. Interchange of active and passive voice.
4. Interchange of affirmative and negative sentence.
5. Changing from interrogative to assertive sentence.
6. Changing exclamatory to assertive sentence.
7. Changing the parts of speech.
8. Changing simple sentence to compound sentence.
9. Changing compound sentence to simple sentence.
10. Changing simple sentence to complex sentence.
11. Changing complex sentence to simple sentence.

2.2.1. Removing an Adverb "too"

This is done by using "**So** ...... **that**"

He is **too** proud to beg. He is **so** proud **that** he cannot beg.
My heart is **too** full for appreciations. My heart is **so** full **that** I cannot accept any more appreciations.
The boy was **too** clever to be caught. The boy was **so** clever **that** he could not be caught.
We are **too** late to catch the bus. We are **so** late **that** we cannot catch the bus.

2.2.2 Changing the Degree of Comparison

Degree of comparison of Adjective and Adverb can be changed without changing the meaning.

Positive degree	Some boys are at least as industrious as Karim.
Comparative degree	Karim is not more industrious than some other boys.
Superlative degree	Karim is not the most industrious boy.
Positive degree	No other man was so strong as Hercules.
Comparative degree	Hercules was stronger than any other man.
Superlative degree	Hercules was the strongest of all men.
Positive degree	Most of the cities in India are not so cool as Dharwad.
Comparative degree	Very few cities in India are cooler than Dharwad.
Superlative degree	Dharwad is one of the coolest cities in India.
Positive degree	No other place I have seen is so beautiful as Darjeeling.
Comparative degree	Darjeeling is more beautiful than any other place I have seen.
Superlative degree	Darjeeling is the most beautiful place I have seen.

2.2.3 Interchange Active and Passive Voice

In active voice .... "Doer of the action is present."
In passive voice ...... "Doer of the action is absent."

Active voice	The people elected him Mayor.
Passive voice	He was elected Mayor by the people.
Active voice	HOD said "I am busy now".
Passive voice	HOD said that he was busy then.
Active voice	Macbeth hoped to succeed Duncan.
Passive voice	It was hoped by Macbeth that he would succeed Duncan.
Active voice	They opened the door.
Passive voice	The door was opened by them.

2.2.4 Interchange Affirmative to Negative Sentence

Affermative	He is literate.
Negative	He is not illiterate.
Active voice	This is all I possess.
Passive voice	I do not possess anything else.
Active voice	Akbar was the greatest of the great Moghuls.
Passive voice	No other great Moghul was so great as Akbar.
Active voice	Everyman makes mistakes sometimes.
Passive voice	There is no man who does not make mistakes sometimes.

2.2.5. Interrogative to Assertive Sentence

Interrogative sentence Assertive sentence	Why worry about what people say? It is foolish to worry about what people say.
Interrogative sentence Assertive sentence	What does it matter whether we win or lose? It matters little whether we win or lose.
Interrogative sentence Assertive sentence	Why waste time in this fruitless occupation? You should not waste time in this fruitless occupation.
Interrogative sentence Assertive sentence	Is this the kind of dress to wear in nursing college? This is not the kind of dress to wear in nursing college.

2.2.6. Exclamatory to Assertive Sentence

Exclamatory sentence Assertive sentence	What a wonderful opportunity! It is a very wonderful opportunity.
Exclamatory sentence Assertive sentence	How kind of you to help him like that! It is very kind of you to help him like that.
Exclamatory sentence Assertive sentence	What a delicious meal! It is a very delicious meal.
Exclamatory sentence Assertive sentence	What a piece of work is man! Man is a wonderful piece of work.

2.2.7. Changing Parts of Speech

I. Replacing NOUN by VERB:

These mangoes have a **sweet smell** but a **sour taste.** These mangoes **smell** sweet but **taste** sour.
He has no **intention** of leaving Dharwad. He **does not intend** to leave Dharwad.

II. Replacing ADVERB by VERB:

They welcomed the good news most **joyfully.** They **rejoiced** most at the good news.
He is **admittedly** the greatest leader of India. It is **admitted** that he is the greatest leader of India.

III. Replacing VERB by NOUN:

Sign this receipt. Affix your **signature** to this receipt.
Acted hastily. His hasty **Act**.

IV. Replacing ADJECTIVE by NOUN:

He was **active.** He was with full of **activity.**
Ant is **intelligent.** Ant has **intelligence.**

V. Replacing NOUN by ADJECTIVE:

Rats gave us **trouble.** Rats were **troublesome** to us.
Wish you the **success** in your deal. He was wished for **successful** deal.

VI. Replacing ADVERB by ADJECTIVE:

In all **probability** the day will be fine. It is quite **probable** that the day will be fine.
Dismiss for the **negligence.** Dismissed for being **negligent.**

VII. Replacing NOUN by ADVERB:

They differ in **essence.** See that they are **essentially** different.
Punishment was **wrong.** He was **wrongly** punished.

VIII. Replacing ADJECTIVE by ADVERB:

Her dress was **poor.** She was **poorly** dressed.
Her dress was **mean.** She was **meanly** dressed.

2.2.8. Simple to Compound Sentence

Simple sentence has one subject and one predicate.

Compound sentence must have two or more coordinate clauses each with subject and predicate.

(Compound Sentence = Double sentence)

Simple sentence Compound sentence	Climbing up the tree, he plucked some mangoes. He climbed up the tree and plucked some mangoes.
Simple sentence Compound sentence	You must work hard to get first prize. You must work hard or you will not win the first prize.
Simple sentence Compound sentence	To everyone's surprise, the project completely failed. The project completely failed and everyone was surprised.
Simple sentence Compound sentence	Owing to drought the crop is short. There is drought and so the crop is short.

2.2.9. Compound to Simple Sentence

This can be done by reducing the number of clauses to one.

Compound sentence Simple sentence	He got up and walked away. Getting up, he walked away.
Compound sentence Simple sentence	He ran away and thus escaped arrest. He ran away in order to escape arrest.
Compound sentence Simple sentence	I called him, but he gave me no answer. In spite of my calling him, he gave me no answer.
Compound sentence Simple sentence	He is rich, yet he is not contented. In spite of his being rich he is not contented.

2.2.10. Simple to Complex Sentence

This is done by expanding a word or phrase into a subordinate clause (say to Noun clause, to Adjective clause or to Adverb clause).

Simple sentence Complex sentence	He liked my **suggestion.** He liked **what I suggested.** (noun clause)
Simple sentence Complex sentence	Tell the **truth.** Tell **what is true.** (noun clause)
Simple sentence Complex sentence	He follows his father's advice. He follows the advice **which was given by his father.** (adjective clause)
Simple sentence Complex sentence	I saw a wounded bird. I saw a bird **that was wounded.** (adjective clause)
Simple sentence Complex sentence	Being sick, he could not work. **As he was sick,** he could not work. (adverb clause)
Simple sentence Complex sentence	He was too dull to understand. **He was so dull that** he could not understand.

2.2.11. Complex to Simple Sentence

This is done by changing Noun clause, Adjective clause and Adverb clause to a word or a phrase.

Complex sentence Simple sentence	He admitted **that he was guilty.** He admitted **his guilt**. (noun clause)
Complex sentence Simple sentence	He asked why I came. He asked the reason for my coming (noun clause)
Complex sentence Simple sentence	I have no money that I can lend you. I have no money to lend you. (adjective clause)
Complex sentence Simple sentence	I saw a man who was blind. I saw a blind man. (adjective clause)
Complex sentence Simple sentence	He was so weak that he could not walk. He was too weak to walk. (adverb clause)
Complex sentence Simple sentence	Whatever you do, I will support. I will support all your acts. (adverb clause)

2.3. SYNTHESIS OF SENTENCES

Following are discussed in this unit:

Synthesis of sentences in terms of simple, compound and complex.

Synthesis of tenses in terms of past, present and future.

Synthesis of speech in terms of direct or indirect.

2.3.1. Combining Sentences

By synthesis we mean "Synthesis of sentences".

Note the following two sentences:

1. The thief heard a shout.
2. The thief ran away.

   When above two sentences are changed (synthesised) to have a look of a single sentence, the sentence will appear as under:

3. Hearing a shout, the thief ran away.

Sentence (1) and (2) are combined into a single sentence in (3) sentence. This process is called "*Synthesis*".

Synthesis is just the opposite of analysis.

Here, we mean the combination of two or more simple sentences into one or new sentence, which could be a:

a. Simple sentence
b. Compound sentence
c. Complex sentence.

2.3.1.1. Simple Sentences to a Simple Sentence

A. By using participle, when sentences have a common subject.

e.g., I read the book.
I returned it to the library.
Having read the book, I returned it to the library.

B. By using the absolute construction, when sentences have different subjects.

e.g., The examination was over.
The college was closed.
The students left for their homes.

The campus looked deserted.

The examination being over, the college being closed and students having left for their homes, the campus looked deserted.

C. By using an infinitive.

e.g., I have some work.

I must do it tonight.

I have some work to do tonight.

D. By using a noun or phrase in apposition.

e.g., Rama defeated Ravana.

Ravana was the King of Srilanka.

Rama defeated Ravana, the king of Srilanka.

E. By using a preposition + a noun or a gerund.

e.g., He had a great deal of influence.

But he could not get the job.

With all his influence he could not get the job.

F. By using an adverb or an adverbial phrase.

e.g., There was an epidemic of gastroenteritis in the village.

The doctor of P.H.C. worked hard.

The doctor had no rest.

He had none to assist him.

During the epidemic of G.E. in the village the doctor worked hard without any rest and with none to assist him.

Examples of synthesis into one simple sentence by using Participles:

Example 1: I received no answer. I knocked a second time.

Receiving no answer, I knocked a second time.

Example 2: A crow stole a piece of cheese. She flew to her nest to enjoy the tasty meal.

Stealing a piece of cheese, a crow flew to her nest to enjoy the tasty meal.

Examples of synthesis into one simple sentence by nouns or phrases in apposition

Example 1: Dr. Abdul Kalam was elected President. He is a well-known scientist.

Dr. Abdul Kalam a well-known scientist was elected President.

Example 2: Pandit Jawaharlal Nehru died in 1964. He was the first Prime Minister of India.

Pandit Jawaharlal Nehru, the first Prime Minister of India, died in 1964.

Examples of synthesis into one simple sentence by prepositions with nouns or gerunds

Example 1: Pravin attended to his duties. He earned promotion.

Pravin earned promotion by attending to his duties.

Example 2: Uma wants to marry a foreigner. Her father is opposed to this.

Uma's father is opposed to her marrying a foreigner.

Examples of synthesis into one simple sentence by nominative absolute construction

Example 1: Rain was plentiful in 2005. Rice is cheap.

Rain having been plentiful in 2005, rice is cheap.

Example 2: Ranadhir fired his arrow. The arrow went high. The tiger sprang on him.

Ranadhir having fired his arrow and the arrow having gone high, the tiger sprang on him.

Examples of synthesis into one simple sentence by infinitives

Example 1: I speak the truth. I am not afraid of it.

I am not afraid of speaking the truth.

Example 2: Drunkard doctor must apologise. He will not escape punishment otherwise.

Drunkard doctor must apologise to escape punishment.

Examples of synthesis into one simple sentence by adverb or adverbial phrases

Example 1: The nurse answered me. Her answer was correct to the question.

The nurse answered me correctly.

Example 2: The manager was obstinate. He refused to listen to the advice.

The manager being obstinate refused to listen to the advice.

Other examples of synthesis into one simple sentence:

Example-1 Homer was a great poet. He was born somewhere. No body knows where. No body knows the birth place of the great poet Homer.
Example-2 Wellington was the greatest of English admirals. Napoleon was the greatest of French soldiers. They were contemporaries. They were the heroes of their respective countries. Wellington, the greatest of English admirals, Napoleon the greatest of French soldiers were contemporary heroes of their respective countries.
Example-3 Rabindranath Tagore founded Shantiniketan. He was a Nobel laureate. He was the author of the National Anthem. Rabindranath Tagore, a Nobel laureate and the author of the National Anthem, founded Shantiniketan.

2.3.1.2. Simple Sentence to Compound Sentence

A compound sentence is one having two or more coordinate clauses. Hence it can be formed only with the help of coordinating conjunctions.

A. By using (Cumulative conjunction) — **and**, **both......... and**, **not only .... but also as well as**

Shankar got up. **He went to the Post Office.**	Shankar got up and went to the Post Office.
She had many friends. **She also had several enemies.**	Not only had she many friends but also several enemies.
Kadakol passed the test. **Kurkuri also passed the test.**	Kadakol as well as Kurkuri passed the test.

B. By using (Adversative conjunction)

but
yet
where as
Nevertheless

Geetha is ill. **She is cheerful.**	Geetha is ill but she is cheerful.
Seetha is rich. **She is miserable.**	Seetha is rich yet miserable.
Tadakod is ambitious. **His brother is quite. the reverse.**	Tadakod is ambitious whereas his brother is quite the reverse.
There was little hope of success **Doctors decided to perform the operation.**	There was little hope of success, nevertheless doctors decided to perform the operation.

C. By using (Alternative conjunction)

or
either .... or
neither .... nor
otherwise
else

You can have cola. You can have tea.	You can have cola or tea.
Venku is a fool. He is a madman.	Venku is either a fool or a madman.
Boss does not smoke. He does not drink.	Boss neither smokes nor drinks.
He will not spend his money. He will not invest it.	He will neither spend his money nor invest it.
You must apologise. You will be punished.	You must apologise otherwise you will be punished.

D. By using (Illative conjunction) **for** **so**

He must be asleep. There is no light in his room.	He must be asleep for there is no light in his room.
He has been working hard. He will get a rank.	He has been working hard so he will get a rank.

A few more examples: (for simple sentences to compound sentence):

Example 1 Football is a vigorous and healthy game. Everybody should play it. Football is a vigorous and healthy game and therefore everybody should play it.
Example 2 Bendre bus was wrecked. No one was hurt. Bendre bus was wrecked, but no one was hurt.
Example 3 The II class carriage is full. We may pay I class fare. We may not travel I class with II class tickets. That is forbidden. The II class carriage being full, we must either pay I class fare or wait for the next train, for we are forbidden to travel in I class with II class tickets.

2.3.1.3 Simple to Complex Sentence

A complex sentence must have a principal clause and one or more subordinate clauses. The subordinate clause may be a Noun clause, an Adjective clause or an Adverb clause.

A. Simple to complex with a noun clause

e.g., Our country stands for peace.
That should be known to everybody.

That India stands for peace should be known to everybody.

OR

It should be known to everybody **that India stands for peace.**

The nurse has failed.

I told her that.

I told the nurse **that she had failed.**

B. Simple to complex with an adjective clause

Here, we use Relative Pronouns as connector of sentence:

who, which, that

e.g., **The attender was caught.**

He had stolen the L.C.D.

The attender **who** had stolen the L.C.D. was caught.

Deepa refused to sing.

Can you tell me the reason?

Can you tell me the reason **why** Deepa refused to sing?

This is an old Fort.

It was built by Kittur Channamma.

This is an old fort that was built by Kittur Channamma.

C. Simple to complex with an adverb clause by connecting with subordinating conjunctions like:

When
As
Since
Till
Where
If
Though
Unless
That
Lest
Whether
Whereas

I went there.

The college was locked.

When I went there, the college was locked.

It may rain.
Then the cricket match will be cancelled.

If it rains, the cricket match will be cancelled.

Ratnam is poor.
He is honest in spite of it.

Though Ratnam is poor, he is honest.

Drakshayani may have gone.
I don't know.

I don't know whether Draksyayani has gone.

Examples of synthesis of complex sentence containing noun clause: (Simple to complex)

He is a sincere worker.
No one can doubt this fact.

No one can doubt the fact that he is a sincere worker.

How did Netaji Subhash Chandra Bose die?
It is a mystery.

It is a mystery how Netaji Subhash Chandra Bose died.

He is a great orator.
This fact cannot be denied.

The fact that he is a great orator cannot be denied.

Who wrote Shakuntala?
Can you tell me that?

Can you tell me who wrote Shakuntala?

Examples of synthesis of complex sentence containing adverb clause: (Simple to complex)

The nurse must be very tired.
She had no sleep last night.

The nurse must be tired, as she had no sleep last night.

He bled profusely.
He died.

As he bled profusely, he died.

Robinson Crusoe discovered the print of a foot on the sand.
He was puzzled.

Robinson Crusoe was puzzled when he discovered the print of a foot on the sand.

We travelled together as far as Florida.
We parted company there.

After we travelled as far as Florida, we parted company.

Examples of synthesis of complex sentence containing adjective clause: (Simple to complex)

The time was four O'clock.
The Bendre bus accident happened then.

The time when Bendre bus accident happened was four o'clock.

The French and Italian languages are different from the Latin language.
Latin was once spoken in almost every part of Europe.

The French and Italian languages are different from the Latin language, which was once spoken in almost every part of Europe.

You are not keeping good health lately.
Can you tell me the reason?

Can you tell me the reason why you are not keeping good health lately?

You put it somewhere.
Show me the place.

Show me the place where you put it.

2.3.2. The Sequences of Tenses

There are 3 main principles. They are:

1. **When the Principal clause is in past tense, the verb in the subordinate clause also should be in the past tense.**

Principal clause	*Subordinate clause*
He **said**	that he **was** not guilty.
He **asked**	whether he **might** go home.
She **was** so weak	that she **could not stand** .

There are two exceptions to above principles:

1. When the subordinate clause expresses a UNIVERSAL TRUTH, it may be put in the present tense, even if the verb in the principal clause is past tense.

   e.g., Copernicus **proved** that the earth **moves** round the sun.
   The Pope **said** that there **is** only one God.
   Gandhi **said** that honesty **is** always the best policy.

2. When the subordinate clause comes after "than" it may be put in any tense required by the context.

   e.g., Kirani shop fellow **demanded** a higher price **than I can pay.**

   In 1900, the value of Rs 1.00 was much greater than it is in 2005 or will be in 2020.

2. When the verb in the principal clause is in the present or future tense, the verb in the subordinate clause may be in any tense that the context requires.

Present Tense
I maintain that he is honest.
I maintain that he was honest.
I maintain that he will be honest.

Future Tense
I shall maintain that he is honest.
I shall maintain that he was honest.
I shall maintain that he will be honest.

3. When the subordinate clause comes after "lest" the only auxiliary verb that it may use is should, whatever be the tense of the verb in the principal clause.

e.g., We start early lest we should miss the train.
We started early lest we should miss the train.
We shall start early lest we should miss the train.

Examples for use of correct tense of verb:

Just as he ________________ the room the clock struck. (to enter)
Just as he **entered** the room the clock struck.

I studied hard in order that I ____________ succeed. (may or might)
I studied hard in order that I **might** succeed.

They erected signposts in order that the road_______ be known.
They erected signposts in order that the road **might** be known.

He begs from door to door that he _______ keep body and soul together.
He begs from door to door that he **may** keep body and soul together.

I come home when it ______ to rain.
I come home when it **ceases** to rain.

I heard that there _________ a disturbance in the city.
I heard that there **was** a disturbance in the city.

2.3.3. Direct and Indirect Speech

Rani said "I want to become a nurse".
Rani said that she wanted to become a nurse.

In first sentence we quote the words of Rani. This is called direct speech. In direct speech we put the words in inverted commas.

In sentence two, we report what Rani said without quoting her exact words. This is called indirect speech.

When we change direct speech to indirect speech, we bring about the following changes:

Comma after said is removed.
Quotation marks are removed.
Conjunction "that" is introduced.
"I" is changed to "she".
"Want" is changed to "wanted".

When we are changing direct speech to indirect speech, we should follow following rules:

1. Present tense of direct speech are changed into corresponding past form in indirect speech.

e.g.,	is	was
	am	was
	are	were
	has	had
	have	had
	can	could
	may	might
	shall	should
	will	would

2. Simple present tense changes to simple past tense:
   He said "I like sweets".
   He said that he liked sweets.
3. Present continuous tense changes into the past continuous:
   Nurse said, "I am buying a new pen".
   Nurse said that she was buying a new pen.
4. Present perfect changes to past perfect.
   Rukmini said "I have read this weekly".
   Rukmini said that she had read that weekly.
5. Present perfect continuous becomes past perfect continuous:
   Professor said "I have been waiting here for a long time".
   Professor said that he had been waiting there for a long time.
6. Past continuous changes to past perfect continuous:
   Mother said "Sudhir was swimming in the pool".
   Mother said that Sudhir had been swimming in the pool.
7. Pronoun and possessive adjective of I and II person in direct speech changes to III person in indirect speech.
   He said "I shall pay your wages tomorrow".
   He said that he would pay his wages the next day.
8. Person addressed reports speech himself, then II person changes to I person.
   He said to me "You alone can save her".
   He told me that I alone could save her.
9. Nearness changes to distance:

this	that
these	those
now	then
here	there
hither	thither
today	that day
tomorrow	the next day
yesterday	the previous day
last night	the night before
ago	before

10. When we change a question to indirect speech, we use **asked, inquired, demanded** etc.
He said "How many brothers have you?"
He asked how many brothers I had.
11. In case of imperative sentences (order, request, warning, advice, command etc.) we use asked, ordered, commanded, requested, implored, advised, warned etc.
"Keep quiet" said the mother to her infant.
The mother asked the infant to keep quiet.
12. In case Exclamations and wishes are present, we use the words like wished, cried out, declared, exclaimed etc.
She said "What a fool Richard is!"
She exclaimed that Richard was a big fool.
13. Interjections and exclamation like Oh!, alas, hurrah etc., we use the words like with delight, with regret, with sorrow etc.
He said "Alas! The poor woman died that very night".
He exclaimed with sorrow that the poor woman died that very night.

Examples of synthesis of Indirect Speech from Direct speech

They wrote "It is time we thought about settling this matter". They wrote that it was time they had thought about settling the matter.
The examiner's orders were, "No one is to bring books into the room nor ask me questions about what I have told you to do". The examiner's orders were that no one was to bring books into the room nor ask him questions about what he had told them to do.
He enquired, "When do you intend to pay me?" He enquired when I intended to pay him.
"Have you anything to say on behalf of the prisoner?" said the judge finally. The judge finally asked whether he had anything to say on behalf of the prisoner.
"Sit down, boys," said the teacher The teacher told the boys to sit down.

	"Hurry up" he said to his servant, "do not waste time". He told his servant to hurry up and not to waste time.
	"How smart you are !" she said. She exclaimed that I was very smart.
	He said, "What a pity you did not come!" He exclaimed that it was a great pity that I had not come.

Conversion of Indirect into Direct Speech

Synthesis or conversions of Indirect Speech to Direct Speech generally do not present any problem.

Examples of conversion of Indirect Speech into Direct Speech:

Indirect Speech	*Direct Speech*
I told him that I had not seen him for months.	"I have not seen him for months", I said to him.
Rama asked Hari if he would change places with him.	Rama said to Hari, "Will you change places with me?"
Abdul said that he had seen that picture.	Abdul said, "I have seen this picture."
The lady inquired if he was now quite well again.	"Are you now quite well again?", the lady inquired.
He ordered him to leave the room and forbade him to return.	He said to me, "Leave the room and do not return."
He advised his sons not to quarrel amongst themselves, when he was dead but to remain united.	He said to his sons, "Do not quarrel among yourselves when I am dead but remain united."

Chapter 3

English Language Usage

3.1. ORDER OF WORDS IN A SENTENCE

In English language inflections are limited. Arrangement of words by putting in an order is of great importance.

Following are specifications in putting the order of a word in sentence formation:

1. Subject comes before verb:
   e.g., **Rama** killed Ravana.
   Nurse undertakes this procedure.
2. Object comes after the verb:
   e.g., The nurse wears **apron.**
   Doctor uses **stethoscope.**
3. When both direct object and indirect object are there, indirect object comes first:
   e.g., Please give **me** your **book.**
   Lend **me** your **ears.**
4. Attributive adjective comes before a noun:
   e.g., Give him **hot** water bath.
   It is a **Royal** sports club.
5. Predicative adjective comes after a noun:
   e.g., The patient is **comatose.**
   The elephant became **wild.**
6. Adjective phrase comes after a noun:
   e.g., He is a man **of words.**
   We travel in a road **of slippery.**
   Go and enjoy the tops **of the mountains.**

7. Adverb is always close to the word it modifies:
   e.g., That man **never** cooks.
   Sister **has just** gone out.

8. Qualifying clauses are attached with qualifying words:
   e.g., Doctor joined the college where he studied.
   Tiger that eats man is dangerous.
9. Alternatives are done to emphasise a point.
   e.g., Quality of Mercy is not strained.
   It droppeth as gentle rain from heaven.

3.2. USE OF CAPITAL LETTERS

Capital letters are used in the following circumstances:

1. At the start of a sentence:
   e.g., Prevention is better than cure.
   Do the sterilisation of instruments.
2. In the start of each line in a poem:
   e.g., Twinkle twinkle little star.
   Oh! I wonder what you are.
3. For names of people, place and river:
   e.g., Arun
   Chennai
   Cauveri.
4. For Nations and Nationality:
   e.g., America
   Americans
   Peru
   Peruvian.
5. For Day, Month, Festival and Historical importance:
   e.g., Sunday
   February
   Deepawavi (Deevali)
   Middle Ages
6. For Books, Play and work of Art:
   e.g., Ramayana
   Taj Mahal
   The Bible
   Mona Lisa

7. For unique things and unique people:
   e.g., Mayor
   Emperor
   King
8. For all adjectives derived from proper noun:
   e.g., Hindu
   Christian
   Biblical
9. For Noun and Pronoun of God and Deity:
   e.g., Lord
   Chinmayananda Ashrama
   Parvathy and Shiva
10. When we write the pronoun 'I':
    e.g., When I approached
    He followed me wherever I went.
11. To write interjection "Oh":
    e.g., He is dead and cremated, Oh! he is dead.
    Cancer, Oh! is he suffering from cancer?

3.3. SPELLING RULES

British (UK English) is standardised for language, spelling, sentence and for expression. But American English (US English), Indian English (Hyderabadi English) have influenced the spelling in English language and much more so in written English. They are accepted in modern English language usage.

UK English	*Other language usage*
Colour	Color, Kolar, Kaulor
Haemoglobin	Hemoglobin, Heemoglobin
Anaemia	Anemia, Aneemia

In UK English certain specific rules are made from the beginning to put the language effectively. These rules are described under spelling usage.

1. 'I' comes before 'e' except (after 'c'). This is relevant when 'ie' or 'ei ' pronounced like 'ee':
   e.g.,

Believe	Conceive
Relieve	Conceit
Achieve	

Grieve
Yield
Field
Receive
Receipt
Device
Deceit
Exceptions are Protein, counterfeit, seize.

2. Words ending 'ee' do not drop 'e':
   e.g.,
   Seeing
   Agreement
3. One syllable word gets doubling of consonant at suffixing vowel:
   e.g.,
   Rob + er = Robber
   Run + ing = Running
4. When last syllable is stressed doubling of consonant occurs:
   e.g.,
   Begin + ing = Beginning
5. 'Y' after consonant changes to 'I':
   e.g.,
   Beautiful
   Carried
   Marriage
   Happily
   Except the words—carrying, marrying, prayed, player, paid and daily.
6. Words ending 'ie' change to 'y' when 'ing' is added:
   e.g.,

Die	Dying
Tie	Tying
Lie	Lying

7. UK English 'l' doubling is common:
   e.g.,
   Travel + er = Traveller
   Signal + ing = Signalling

8. Words where second 'l' is dropped when 'ful' is added:
   e.g.,
   Skilful
   Wilful
9. When 'e' is silent at the end of word, they get dropped when they are joined with word beginning with vowel:
   e.g.,
   Hope + ing = Hoping
   Drive + er = Driver
10. Special cases where 'e' is retained:
   e..g.,

Charge	Chargeable
Courage	Courageous

3.4 PROPER USAGE OF VERB

A. When you use verb it must agree with:
   Its subject
   Its number
   and with its person
   otherwise you may end up with **"error proximity"**.
   e.g., Today number of OT cases **was** not high.
   Use of snack, tea, soft drinks, food, salad and other eatables **has** not been without some effect.
   The results of diet therapy and nutritional therapy **are** slow outcome.
   The conduct and behaviour of Pinto, Harry and Rosy **were** not good.
   The children **were** frightened
   Mr. Sudhir **is** coming.

B. By joining singular noun or pronoun we use plural verb.
   e.g., Ward nurse and staff **are** coming.
   Are your brother and sister at hostel?
   Nurse and I **were** playing.

C. If one idea is written it takes singular verb.
   e.g., My only breakfast **is** bread and butter.
   The politician and Minister **is** dead.
   Honour and glory **is** his military reward.

D. When subject is joined with 'with', 'as well as', it shall come in singular.

e.g., The TV with its appendages **was** given warrantee.

The boat with its boarders **was** lost.

Court in its judgement **allows** justice as well as mercy.

E. More singular subjects when connected with 'or' 'nor' it is used in singular.

e.g., In searching for lost ring no nook and corner **was** left behind.

When you go to desert, neither food nor water **is** available.

F. When two plural subjects connected with 'or', 'nor' verb must be plural.

e.g., Neither the rings nor bangles **were** found.

Either foods or water **are** available in desert.

G. When different persons are referred verb should agree with nearer subject.

e.g., Either doctor or nurse **is** mistaken

Neither the nurse nor the doctor **is** to be blamed.

H. Use singular verb when you are using the following:

Either
Neither
Each
Everyone
Many a

e.g., Each of the instruments **is** useful.

Everyone of the wards **is** full.

Many a nurse **has done** so.

I. When you use 'each', 'every', to qualify nouns use singular verbs:

(in spite of your using 'and')

e.g., Every male and female patient **was** given free clothes and fruits.

J. When nouns are plural, but are singular in meaning, they take singular verb.

e.g., The news of one lakh deaths by earthquake **is** true.

Mathematics **is** one of the optionals in science.

K. Pains and means take both singular and plural when construction of sentences are made.

e.g., Great pains **have been taken** by mother in her delivery.

Much pains **has been taken** by mother in her delivery.

To save that patient all possible means **have been taken.**

The means employed to save the patient **is** okay.

L. When 'income' is meant by the word 'means' it takes plural verb.

e.g., Rich man's means **are** ample.

Her means **are** very much on lower side.

M. When 'nouns' are singular, but mean plural, they take up plural verb.

e.g., At Present Infosys share rate, 100 shares **cost** 5 lakh rupees.

Doctors fee, nowadays **are** costing more.

N. 'None' a singular word takes plural verb.

e.g., None of the tutors **are** OK here.

O. In case of collective noun, if collective noun is considering 'one', use singular verb. If collective noun is considering 'more than one' use plural verb.

e.g., The Kartar Singh Committee **gives** MPWs report.

The college council committee **are** divided on the issue at the meeting.

P. Plural nouns when depict single object or single unit, use singular verb.

e.g., United States **has** a big Navy.

The Arabian Nights **is** a great favourite.

Q. While using plural nouns for specific quantity use singular verb.

e.g., Two hours **is** allowed to each guest speaker.

Five hundred miles **is** a long distance.

3.5. PROPER USAGE OF NOUN AND PRONOUN

A. Note the following countable nouns and pronouns.
Pen, Book, Orange etc.
These countable nouns and pronouns can have plural and can be used with 'a' or 'an':

Pens	a pen
Books	a book
Oranges	an orange

B. Note the following uncountable nouns and pronouns. These uncountable nouns and pronouns cannot have plural and cannot be used with 'a' or 'an':
News
Furniture
Business
Information

C. Uncountable thing can be made to a unit in expression:
A piece of news
A portion of information

D. Possessive case is used for living things:
Nature's law
President's security

E. Possessive case in stereotyped phrases as under:
For God's sake.
For goodness' sake.

F. Possessive case in nouns of space and time is allowed:
In a month's time.
An hour's work.

G. Possessive case if has two nouns add apostrophe s ('s) to last noun:
My wife, Deputy commissioner's office,
Her son, Inder's ring.

H. When a noun is qualified by two possessive cases, both should have possessive signs:
Doctors' and nurses' quarters.
Marie's and Nestlé's biscuits.

I. When a noun is qualified by two possessive cases, and if they have joint possession, the latter will have the possessive sign:

The husband and wife's quarrel has come to an end.
Son and daughter's property is distributed.

J. Object of a verb or object of a preposition when is a pronoun, it should be in objective form.
Let this be between you and me.
Our tenants have given trouble to my father and me.

K. A pronoun after 'than' or after 'as' is usually objective case.
My wife is taller than me.
I read better than him.
Raghu is as tall as her.

L. Pronoun must agree with number, gender and person.
Air passengers must allow the check of **their** luggage.
Every student should bring **his** own plate.

M. When we use any of the following words, like:
Anybody
Everybody
Everyone
Anyone
Each
Gender is used according to the context.
e.g., I help everyone of my nursing students in her studies.

N. If back reference is there for a pronoun for 'every body', 'every one', 'each' etc., use masculine gender.
Any body can eat this if he likes.
Everyone ran as fast as he could.

O. If you are using indefinite pronoun 'one', use it throughout even repeatedly. (present grammar suggests to avoid such usage)
One should not boast of one's own success.

P. None can be singular or plural as per context.
Did you buy any golden bangles? There were none in the market.
Have you brought me a telegram? There was none for you.

Q. Use 'anyone' when more than two people or more than two things are considered.
Roopa is more beautiful than anyone of her three sisters.

R. 'Each', 'either' and 'neither' should have singular verb.
Each of the nurses **has done** well in examination.
Either of the operations **leads to** good survival rate.
Neither of the tutors **was invited** to the party.

S. When you are using, note the following words:
Who = Nominative
Whom = Objective
e.g., **Who** these girls are I really don't know.
Nurse **whom** you thought clever has failed in the examination.

T. Subject of a verb is relative pronoun. Then see that verb agrees in number and person with the antecedent of the relative pronoun.
e.g., She is one of the intelligent girls that **have** passed through this school of nursing.
(Here, antecedent of that is **'girls'** and **not 'one'**)

U. 'And which' can be used as conjunction to join two relative clauses to the same antecedent.
e.g., Heggadeji possessed a 400 years old door **which** was of excellent workmanship **and which** has been in his family for generations.

3.6. PROPER USE OF ADJECTIVES

i. To express quality, adjective is used with a verb:
e.g., Doctor feels **happy.**
The scent smells **pungent.**

ii. In grammatical use, 'kind' and 'sort' take up 'these' or 'those'.
e.g., Those **kind** of furniture.

iii. Adjectives like senior, junior, superior, inferior, anterior, posterior etc., take 'to' instead of 'than'.
e.g., Mother Superior is **senior to** that mother.
King died **prior to** 1942 war.

iv. During comparison of two things, comparative degree is preferred.
e.g., This scalpel is the **better** of the two.
Ranga is the **taller** of the two.

v. When comparison follows 'than', the compared thing must be excluded by using 'other'.

e.g., She is **weaker than** other women living.
Gandhiji has done more for the **unity** of India **than** any other man.

vi. At superlative comparison, latter term should include former.
e.g., Of all the women she is the **most beautiful.**
Ganga is the **largest of all** rivers in India.

vii. Avoid double comparison and superlatives. It was common in Shakespearean English.

viii. 'Preferable' should follow 'to' and not 'more preferable'.

ix. Older, oldest ...... are said of persons.
Elder, eldest .... refer to family members.

x. Always use "first two" and not "two first".

xi. Remember Few is negative.
A few is positive.

xii. Remember "Little" is not much.
A little is some.

xiii. Use the word "Oral" and not "Verbal" in written and vocabulary English.

3.7. PROPER USE OF VERBS

i. Subject should have a verb. And verb should agree with its subject.

ii. Single verb in a compound sentence:
e.g., Not a dish was served, not a tea.

iii. Differentiate the following words:
Lay (Transitive followed by object).
Lie (verb intransitive, no object).

iv. Present participle not used for action which is not contemporaneous with the action of main verb.
President left Delhi on Saturday and arrived there on Monday. (do not use arriving there)

v. Wrong usage of verb with 'to' infinitive.

Wrong usage	*Correct usage*
He learns to swim	He learns swimming
To avoid meeting	Avoids meeting
Missed to see	Missed seeing

vi. Wrong usage of verb with 'about', 'for'.

Wrong usage	*Correct usage*
Discussed about	Discussed
Described about	Described
Ordered for	Ordered
Requested for	Requested

3.8. PROPER USAGE OF ADVERB

i. Adverb should be placed in proper position to get clear meaning. It is advisable to put adverb to the word which it modifies:
   Johnson went almost to the top when he died.
ii. 'Only' should be put before the word which the adverb modifies:
   He ate only two idlis.
iii. When you use 'ever', 'never' and 'scarcely', they should follow verb:
   He remembers ever.
   He remembers never.
   He remembers scarcely.
iv. When you make affirmation, use double negative:
   I haven't got any latest journals.
   Husband could not see any wit in his wife.
v. Adjectives should not be used for adverbs:
   Do not use 'quicker' or 'dear'.
   Instead use 'more quickly' or 'pay dearly' etc.
vi. In case of usage of 'never', 'ever', note the following dictum:
   Seldom or never is allowed.
   Seldom if ever is allowed.
   Seldom or ever is not allowed.
vii. Do not use 'that' as an adverb. Use always 'so':
   Nurse went only so far. (not *that for*)
   Wife was so angry that she slammed her husband. (not *wife was that angry*)
viii. Use the word 'too' to give meaning of **more than enough:**
   It should not be used instead of 'very' or instead of 'much'.
   Too good
   Too full
   Too much

ix. 'Of course' should be used when we mean **inevitable.** Does the nurse do the nursing well? Certainly she does.
(do not use *not 'of course she does'* which is wrong).

3.9. PROPER USE OF CONJUNCTION

i. Presently we are not using *except* as a conjunction in place of *unless:*
I shall not operate unless you ask me.
(not *except you ask me*)
ii. Using *without* as conjunction is not good.
I shall not pass you unless you study.
(not *without study* which is wrong).
iii. *Like* cannot be used as conjunction.
She sings as her mother.
(not *like her mother*)
iv. *Directly* cannot be used as conjunction. In this circumstance, ***as soon as*** is preferred.
As soon as session of parliament commenced, the Government was pressed to do something for the employed.
v. Redundant use of conjunction *that* is avoided.
vi. Scarcely should be followed by 'when'.
Scarcely had official put the money in purse, when vigilance squad caught him. (*than vigilance squad caught* is wrong)
vii. 'No sooner' should be followed by 'than'. Don't use 'but'.
viii. Use **seldom or never.** Don't use **seldom or ever.**
ix. **Neither** should follow **nor** and *never or.*

3.10. COMMON IDIOMS

Idioms are expressions peculiar to any language. They play important role in flowering the language.

Absence of mind = Obstruction of thought.

From A to Z = Completely or thoroughly.

Usually we have seen that verb is followed by preposition to form an idiom.

Dispose of

Call in

Usually we have seen that verb is followed by an adverb to form an idiom.

Come about

Set aside

Idioms in Usage

To go about	To move from place to place
To live above one's means	To spend more than income
Abundance of the heart	Overflowing emotion
To put it across	To get even with
Act of God	Untoward happenings
Ad hoc	Formed for one subject only
To bid adieu	To take leave
To look after	To take care of
A golden age	A prosperous period
To run amuck	To run about madly killing people indiscriminately
To do away with	To make an end of anything
To make away with	To kill
To bear with	To tolerate
To beat about the bush	Approach in a round about way
To bell the cat	To lead in dangerous work
Between cup and lip	Between hope and reality
Birds of the same feather	Persons of similar habits
Bit a bit	Gradually
Black and white	In writing
Once in a blue moon	Rarely
Bolt from the blue	Full surprise
Born with silver spoon	Born in a rich family
Bread and butter	Livelihood
Make a clean breast of	Confess
Build castle in the air	Plan impossible scheme
Burn one's finger	To suffer
Feather in the cap	Something to be proud of
Put cart before the horse	Reverse natural order
Chip of the same block	Same
Cock and bull story	Unbelievable story
Give a deaf ear	Disregard
Blessing in disguise	Misfortune which produce a good result
Go to dogs	Ruined
Give one's ear	To attend
Come to an end	Become exhausted
To catch the eye of some one	To attract the attention of somebody

In good faith	With sincerity
To feel the pulse	To find out one's secret opinion
To cut a sorry figure	To be ridiculed
To make a fortune	To earn a lot
From hand to mouth	To live within a little income
To get rid of	To leave
To kill the goose that lays golden eggs	To sacrifice future profits
Heart to heart	Frank and free
At helm of affairs	Those who control or are in authority
To play hide and seek	To deceive
Jack of all trades	One who can do all things
To win laurels	To win honours
Lean year	Famine
To pull one's leg	To deceive
To read between the lines	To catch the secret meaning
Man in the moon	Very rare person
Once in a blue moon	Now and then
The naked truth	Truth without trimmings
Nip in the bud	To check growth of
To pass away	To die
Penny wise and pound foolish	To serve a low cost thing at the cost of very costly thing
Out of question	Not worth discussing
To reap the fruit of	To enjoy the consequences of
The rules of the road	Etiquette
A rolling stone gathers no moss	A person who changes his profession too often is generally unsuccessful
Out of senses	Mad
To cut a sorry figure	To be subjected to shame
Wear and tear	Damage sustained as a result of ordinary use
A man of word	Who keeps promise
To eat humble pie	Apologise
To eat your words	Go back from promise
Won his laurel	Acquired glory
Turned a deaf ear	Disregarded
By hook or by crook	By any means
Off and on	Occasionally
On and off	At intervals
Made up my mind	Decided
In the long run	Ultimately
Brought to light	Disclosed
Burnt his finger	Got into trouble

Wash my hands	Not to involve
Keep in touch	Have intimate knowledge
True to their salt	Faithful
Smell a rat	Suspect
Took him to task	Reproved
Every inch	Completely
Caught red handed	Held at committing theft
Cut him short	Interrupt
Thrust your nose into	Meddle
Right hand man	Most efficient
Upto the mark	Excellent
In hot water	In trouble

3.11. FIGURES OF SPEECH

When we speak by departing from ordinary form of expression, we start using figures of speech.

We use words which give resemblance to what normally or in ordinary way we speak. The common figures of speech which are:

Simile
Metaphor
Personification
Apostrophe

We speak ironically by using word which gives opposite meaning. It is called irony.

We use questioning not to get answer but to point out effectively. This is called interrogation.

To draw attention we use exclamation.

Series of ideas used in stepladder manner is called climax.

3.11.1. Simile

If two words have at least one point in common, simile is used to compare them. Same kind of comparison is not simile.

Love is like red rose.
As proud as peacock.

3.11.2. Metaphor

It is an implied simile. When metaphor is used it takes the things for granted as if two are one.

Love is rose.
He was peacock in pride.

3.11.3. Personification

Here nonliving things are considered living by giving life.

Death lays his hand on every man on this earth.
Pride always rides on a horse.

3.11.4. Apostrophe

We speak and address on an object which is not there or we address a dead person, we use apostrophe.

Yamaraja, where are you?
Liberty has killed every body.

3.11.5. Irony

Here real meaning is told by opposite word.

Brutus was an honourable man.
Lion shows mercy on him.

3.11.6. Exclamation

Exclamation used to draw attention at talk.

How gigantic his personality is!
What a piece of computer human brain is!

3.11.7. Climax

Put dialogue with series of ideas which will build up in the order of importance.

Karna in Mahabharat was a hero like Arjun, a strong man like Bheema, a Satyawadi like Dharmaraya.

Nurse is noble in reason, fantastic in procedures and an angel in protection.

Chapter 4

Pattern of Verb

By pattern of verb we mean "the structure of verb in common usage". There are some basic verb patterns in day-to-day literary usage as well as conversational usage.

In traditional grammar, we come across 20 different patterns which are as under:

Pattern No.	*Pattern of verb*
1.	**Subject + verb** Baby + cries
2.	**Subject + verb + subject complement** That + is + a stethoscope
3.	**Subject + verb + direct object** We + should treat + the patient
4.	**Subject + verb + indirect object + direct object** The tutor + gave + us + problem solving exercises
5.	**Subject + Verb + Direct Object + Preposition + Prepositional Object** The tutor + gave + problem solving exercise + to + all of us
6.	**Subject + verb + noun/pronoun + adjective** She + likes + her pen + green
7.	**Subject + verb + preposition + prepositional object** The nurse + complained + of + tutor's rudeness
8.	**Subject + verb + 'to' infinitive** Doctor + wants + to operate
9.	**Subject + verb + noun/pronoun + 'to' infinitive**
	The nurse + ordered + the patient + to close her eyes

Contd.

Contd.

10.	**Subject + verb + gerund** The child + enjoys + reading comics
11.	**Subject + verb + noun/pronoun + present participle** You + keep + the operation + going
12.	**Subject + verb + noun/pronoun + plain infinitive** We + saw + her + coming in
13.	**Subject + verb + noun/pronoun + past participle** Tutor + wants + this figure + written
14.	**Subject + verb + noun/pronoun + (to be) complement** The Dean + appointed + her + (to be) Matron of hospital
15.	**Subject + verb + that-clause (object of the verb)** The teacher + hopes + (that) you would pass
16.	**Subject + verb + noun/pronoun + that-clause** Raja Ramanna + warned + the leader + that there were bombs in the crowd.
17.	**Subject + verb + interrogative + clause** I + wonder + what + the nurse wants
18.	**Subject + verb + noun/pronoun + interrogative + clause** Can + you tell + the doctor + where + it pains?
19.	**Subject + verb + interrogative + to infinitive** Student + didn't + know + how to give enema
20.	**Subject + verb + noun/pronoun + interrogative + to infinitive** I + shall show + the students + how to give enema

Let us illustrate four common verb patterns.

4.1. SIMPLE VERB

When a sentence contains subject and a verb and can give full meaning, we call it simple verb.

e.g., Birds fly
Dogs bark
Fire burns
Time flies

4.2. VERB WITH SUBJECT COMPLEMENT

The sentence contains a noun along with a subject complement.

e.g.,
He is an engineer.
They are our neighbours.
Those are our fields.
The play was superb.

4.3. VERB WITH DIRECT OBJECT

The verb will be a transitive verb when it has an object. The normal order of words in an English sentence is:

Subject + verb + Direct object

e.g.,
The tutor punished the nurse.
Pratap Singh likes sword.
I know her house.
Mary closed the window.

4.4. VERB WITH NOUN COMPLEMENT

By using common verbs like elect, appoint, call, make or choose, the pattern will have:

Subject + verb + noun/pronoun + noun complement

e.g.,
Doctor considered the treatment (to be) unwise.
He called her (to be) a fool.
The commission reported Lava (to be) a punishable criminal.
I do not consider the plan (to be) wise.

Chapter 5

Question Tags

Communication in man is not brief. It extends to repetition. Common practice is that man makes assertion, deduces statements and again starts asking questions. Asking questions are, no doubt, for confirmation.

The way of making a statement followed by a Question by man in conversation is called **Question Tags.**

e.g., Patient is crying with pain. **Is he not?**

Massive heart attack kills man. **Isn't it?**

Keep distance from infectious cases. Otherwise you get infection. **Don't you?**

Sister, you are busy. **Are you?**

Above underlined phrases contain pronoun and never a noun. So subject of the **question tag** is always a pronoun.

Note few more question tags.

There are some married nursing students in your class. Aren't there?

Nurse, I am alright. Am I not ?

Doctor, please wait a minute. Can you?

Ward nurse and Matron called me to attend an emergency case. Haven't they?

Notice the following question Tag:

You will do it. Won't you?

This can be said in two ways. If you say it with the voice falling on "do it and won't you, it means.

'I am sure, you will do it. I think I can depend upon your doing it'.

But, if you say it with the voice rising on "won't you"? It becomes a query.

'I think you will do it, but I am not quite sure, please tell me if I am wrong.'

Similarly see the following Question Tags:

He will come today. Won't he?

You won't disappoint us. Will you?

The train is arriving on time. Isn't it?

You can help us. Can't you?

It is worth the trouble. Isn't it?

We could do with another fan. Couldn't we?

He shouldn't have lost his temper. Should he?

In the above question tags you can notice that when the statement is POSITIVE, the tag question is NEGATIVE and when the statement is NEGATIVE , the tag question is POSITIVE.

5.1 SHORT ANSWERS

In reply to question, one has to give answer. They are verbal questions and hence one has to give short answers to continue other dialogues. Any short answer will carry:

1. 'Yes' or 'No'.
2. A pronoun.
3. An auxiliary.

Let us give short answers to above mentioned questions:

Question Tag	*Short Answers*
There are some married nursing students in your class. Aren't there?	Yes. There are.
Nurse, I am alright. Am I not?	No. You aren't.
Doctor, please wait a minute. Can you?	Yes. I can.
Ward nurse and Matron called me to attend an emergency case. Haven't they?	Yes. They have (called).

Some additional short answers:

Can you drive motorbike? No I can't.

Did your colleague nurse say anything? No she didn't.

5.2 AGREEMENT AND DISAGREEMENT IN CONVERSATION

In reply to Question Tag we have to give affirmative statements, which is 'Yes' OR 'No'. They are called 'Agreement' or 'Disagreement' respectively.

Usual words used are:

Yes
So
Of course
No
Oh! No
Oh! Yes

e.g., Giving enema is a good nursing procedure.

Answer: Yes it is.

Patient has severe spasmodic cough. He can't help coughing.

Answer: Yes. He has (cough).
No he can't (help it).

I suppose you know assisting Tonsillectomy operation.

Answer: No. I don't (know).

In chemistry laboratory you broke the beaker at experiment.

Answer: Oh! No. I didn't (break).

I didn't break it.

Answer: Oh! But you did.

5.3 ADDITIONS TO REMARKS

There are four types of additions in our conversation.

A. Affirmative assertion to affirmative remarks.
Nursing superintendent was late for the meeting. So were you.
Asha likes oranges. So do I.

B. Negative additions to negative remarks.
Asha doesn't like oranges. Nor do I.
I cannot diagnose the illness. Nor can my tutor.

C. Negative additions to affirmative remarks.
Nurse knows the procedure. But I don't.
I can do L.P. (lumbar puncture). But my colleague can't.

D. Affirmative additions to negative remarks.
She cannot operate. But I can.
Tutor doesn't know sister Kamat. But Matron does.
Radha didn't see movie "Taal". But Gopi did.

Thus, Question Tag, Short Answers, Agreements and Disagreements in Conversation and Additions to remarks are STRUCTURES in Literary and Conversational component in English language.

Chapter 6

Written Composition

Writing is an Art to communicate ideas and feelings of a person to others. Good writing is hallmark of good communication. The writer should be writing with a accuracy, appropriateness and attentiveness. The brevity and brightness of a write up should awaken the reader. Added to all these the write up must be with proper use of grammar to give consistent and concrete flow of thought.

Different kinds of writing are:

1. Paragraph writing
2. Story writing
3. Poem writing
4. Letter writing
5. Précis writing
6. Passage explanations
7. Essay writing
8. Autobiography writing
9. Dramatic dialogue writing
10. Review writing
11. Para phrasing
12. Writing at work
13. Writing at home
14. Writing at college
15. Writing applications
16. Notes writing
17. Article to journals.

6.1. PARAGRAPH WRITING

This refers to a write up of a Para by selecting a topic through composition of number of sentences as a group.

When related sentences are written they automatically develop to a single topic of importance.

Grammatically even one sentence can be a Para. But eventually to depict an idea we need to write unlimited number of sentences which go to form a Para.

Following criteria are maintained in the write up of paragraph. They are:

1. There must be one idea in a paragraph. This is called unity of thought.
2. Sequence of write up must be logically arranged which is called 'an order of write up construction'.
3. The write up should have different pattern of sentences to avoid monotony.

Examples of Paragraphs

It is the winter of discontent in Kerala *Kalamandalam*, an institution founded by the great poet *Vallathol Narayana Menon* in 1930 to bring about a revival of Kerala's classical arts. The cultural colossus of Kerala, which revived many stagnant art forms including *Kathakali, Mohiniyattom, Koodiyattom, Panchavadyam* and *Thullal,* and produced many stalwarts, is now facing an existential crisis of sorts.

(introducing Kerala Kalamandalam by Journalist R. Gopakumar)

The myth of modern man does not do away with the truth that man always remains essentially the same with regard to his moral obligation, his need of redemption and the true coarseness of happiness. Man, as such, always lacks of some positive good. He always lacks of something required for an adequate adjustment and efficiency. Man is complex and needs many things.

(Care for your basic needs—from HOW TO USE PERSONAL EFFICIENCY by J Maurus)

This too was duly acknowledged but I was surprised to find some currency notes in the envelope along with his letter.

"Madam" he had written, "It is kind of you to have sent me money for the next six months. But I was not in Bellary for the last two months. One month, our college was on holiday and during the next month, there was a strike. So I stayed at home for those two months. My expenditure during these months was less than Rs. 300 per month.

Therefore, I am sending you the Rs. 300 that I have not used for the last two months. Kindly accept this amount."

I was taken aback. Such poverty and yet such honesty!

('Honesty comes from the heart' from "wise and otherwise a salute to life" by Sudha Murthy)

O strong and Omnipresent God! Vouchsafe, we beseech Thee, the grace to approach Thee always and everywhere in Thy Glory—Thee, Who hast no equal—and under all circumstances to take refuge in Thee.

('Faith in God' from Sama Veda 2209)

Dread the day wherein one soul shall not make satisfaction for another soul, neither shall many intercession be accepted from the, nor shall any compensation be received, neither shall they be helped.

('Judgement' from Koran II)

Few people realise that Christianity came to India as early as the first century after Christ, long before Europe turned to it, and established a firm hold in South India.

('Church in India' an Autobiography by Pandit Jawaharlal Nehru)

This volume does not purport to be the contemporary history of the nation during my term as President of India (1987-1992). It deals only with matters with which I had been connected in one form or another. There were several issues of national importance in which the President of India was not involved and they do not find a place in these pages.

(Prologue by R.Venkataraman in his "My Presidential Years")

The word nurse has come from the word nourishing, which means tending and helping all who need it, especially the sick. Her adequate service depends upon her understanding the mind and body of other individual in her skills used in nursing profession.

(from 'Sociology for Nurses' by Dr.G.N. Prabhakara)

Population education is a health education programme which provides for a study of population situation in the community, country and world with the purpose of developing rational and responsible attitude among present generation towards family planning behaviour.

('Population Education' in Text Book of Community Health for Nurses by Dr.G.N. Prabhakara).

6.2. STORY WRITING

Story writing requires practice. This was used for narrating a tale in ancient times. With total plot in our mind we can write a good story, by arrangement in sequence.

Criteria for good story writing:

1. Ariel view or a plot in mind is a requisite.
2. Sequence must be made natural and not artificial.
3. Continuity should be maintained.
4. In between we can use conversations to make it be real one.
5. Surprises are maintained in the sequences.
6. Title of the story given should be from main incident or main character.
7. Simple language makes the story bright.

Example of Story Writing

Detective Rama

Rama and Krishna were good friends. Rama's father had a business, whereas Krishna's parents were not well off. They were skilled labourers and earned livelihood by working hard. Rama was not good at studies, but was fond of becoming a detective. Rama used to read detective books and used to watch detective serials.

Krishna's birthday was round the corner. Rama was planning to give a gift to his friend. He decided to give him a tape recorder.

The selected tape recorder was light weighted, smaller in size and was of a superb quality to record faintest sound from a distance.

"Lalitha, we will put the cassette and put it on recording mode at present", Rama told his sister.

"But why in recording mode?", enquired Lalitha.

"Later we can replay the recordings and listen to who was saying what all things", explained Rama.

"You are fantastic", said Lalitha smilingly.

Rama packed the tape recorder and started moving out of the house, when the phone rang up.

"Rama, this is Harry. Please come to Golden Park in front of your house. I want to talk to you secretly for 10 minutes. It is urgent", said Harry over phone.

Rama and Harry had discussions for 10 minutes. Suddenly Rama remembered that the tape recorder with cassette is on. He re-winded and played the tape recorder.

"Tomorrow we meet at State Bank at 11 AM sharp, we will rob the bank", came the voice with lot of disturbances.

Rama guessed that this sound must have been from somebody in the park. Immediately he went to police station and informed the sub-inspector of the station.

"Good, we will be at Bank with police force to nab them", sub-inspector told Rama and thanked him for his detective sense.

At the dot of time, police force was there and in a flash of a second, police locked the main gate of the bank and sealed the route for robbers. They pounced upon them and overpowered them.

"Move", police pushed the robbers to police van.

Next day this was the main item in the newspaper. Bank rewarded Rama Rs.1001/- and a certificate for his help.

All were happy in helping the arrest of the robbers at the bank.

"Congrats Mr. Detective Rama", Krishna greeted.

6.3. PRÉCIS WRITING

This is from 18th century French word meaning 'summary of the text' or 'an abstract'.

Précis writing is an art of expressing the write up in a few words. In other words writing main or essential points constitutes précis writing.

Précis writing doesn't have detailing at any point of time.

Criteria for good précis writing are:

1. Write up should be made an experience in life.
2. Write up should give clear and concise facts.
3. Make it practicable to use in life for accurate expression.
4. Read a passage, catch main points, summarise without comments.
5. Revise if necessary.

Example of Précis Writing

The Art of Poetry

Richard Aldington

What is the purpose of poetry in modern life? Let us begin by saying what it is not, obviously, the purpose is not ethical. The poet does not desire to improve the morals of his readers. The old cant of a poet's "message" is now completely discredited and the theory of "uplift" may be left to the unimportant provinces where it still flourishes. Didactic poetry is now almost universally recognised as impertinence.

The danger of poetry's becoming a kind of after dinner amusement is far greater than the danger of its reverting to a method of moral instruction. Literature today is too cheap; poetry tends to become a sort of pleasant little hobby, something which nice people play with when there is nothing more amusing to do. People's minds are absorbed in commerce, sociology and politics. Literature has lost its prestige. We are very far from the times when Loren O Valla's discoursing on Latin grammar disturbed the supremacy of the Popes and equally far from the more recent times when a pamphlet by Chatenbriand re-established, at least temporarily, the dynasty of the Bourbons. Literature seems out of touch with men's lives, their real interests. And so in their popular forms, books are something people read to amuse themselves to beguile a tedious railway journey, or to pass the long unemployed Sunday afternoon. Knowledge of modern literature, even in its more intellectual forms and especially poetry is an accomplishment not a passion; an entertainment for idle women not a real force.

Petrarch who wept with emotion over the copy of Homer he could not read would appear a very ridiculous sight today. Nobody would think of becoming emotional over the possession of a mere book, an object to amuse a few leisure hours. I do not suppose many read modern poetry for mere amusement; but even here the motive is not so much a purely aesthetic enjoyment as sort of snobbery, an outcome either of the foolish desire to know the latest fashion in poets or of that affection of superior wisdom which claims a monopoly of culture.

It describes the purpose of poetry in modern life. It is not for leisure hours. It is an accomplishment. Petrarch's emotional weeping on copy of Homer is ridiculous sight today. People do not read for aesthetic enjoyment or for becoming wise and cultured.

6.4. ESSAY WRITING

Essay literally means "an attempt" to express thoughts on a given topic which is different from a treatise which is an elaborate write up.

It can be defined as a piece of prose composition, generally written, in short form, on any selected topic.

According to Dr. Johnson an essay is "a loose sally of the mind" a sensitive form of self-expression. To write an essay, specialised skill is needed.

Try to learn this literary composition on a topic of your choice.

Different types of essays are:

1. **Descriptive essay:** Simple, gives description.
   e.g., The Taj Mahal.
   Visit to Zoo Garden.
   Niagara Falls.
2. **Narrative essay:** Narrates the incident.
   e.g., Tsunami.
   A short light.
   The boyhood of Gandhi.
3. **Reflective essay:** Thoughts or reflections.
   e.g., Social custom.
   The purpose of living.
   Courage.
4. **Imaginative essay:** Imaginations.
   e.g., I am a Naya Paisa.
   If I were a millionaire.
   Lilliputian adventure.
5. **Expository essay:** Expound theory.
   e.g., Rebirth.
   Nature's cure.
   Evolution of man.

Characteristics of the Essay

- An essay will have.
  a. A beginning (An introduction)
  b. A middle (Body)
  c. An end (Conclusion).
- An orderly development of thought from para to para.
- Adaptation of style to and treatment of the topic.
- Illustration and anecdotes are used.

Hints for Essay Writing

1. Have an idea, analyse the situation before writing.
2. Write down all your thoughts, later you can select only applicable ones.
3. Arrangement should be under different heads.
4. Give brief and striking introduction to the essay.
5. Plan and write an appropriate body.
6. Give forceful and effective conclusion.

Suggestions for BEGINNING (Introduction) and ENDING (Conclusion)

Beginning (Introduction)	*Ending (Conclusion)*
Abrupt opening without introduction	With brief summary
Start with definition	With a prediction
Begin with anecdote	With a quotation
Begin with a quotation	With an interrogative remark
Begin with a question	
Begin with a proverb	
Begin with vivid description	

Examples of Essays

Health is Wealth

Positive health and 'person years' in good health has been the symbol of the progress of a person, his family and his society. Health is the most important wealth of man. If man is gifted with good health, it is great to get the gift from the creator of the man. When man is healthy, he can gain wealth, education, job, property. All are secondary to health. If he succumbs to ill health, he cannot enjoy physical wealth or physical pleasures.

Not long ago, man was of the opinion that the disease is caused by the curse of God. In illness, man used to offer prayers and poojas instead of medicine. In those days modern medicine was not developed and there was no qualified doctors to treat illness. Herbs and local native medicine used to score over other methods of treatment. This used to be the reason for higher death rates including mothers and children in the community.

Today we have found out the germs that cause illness in man. Man has discovered drugs for infections and even non-infectious diseases. Health is maintained by different modes of intervention. Preventive, curative and rehabilitative care has changed the positive health status of man in the universe. Present strategies have changed the morbidity and mortality in terms of reduced maternal mortality, infant mortality and death rates.

Health is not only physical health, it also includes mental health, social health and spiritual health of man. Now, health awareness has spread all over man's activities. Physical games, sports are given importance for positive health of children and adult. Government, through many agencies launched National Health Programmes giving health care to all sector of the community. Awareness is created through AIR, DD. In school curriculum science lessons are included which depicts the keeping of good health.

Since infectious person is dangerous in spreading disease to other, measures are taken through surveillance, quarantine to contain such diseases. It is the duty of citizen to keep good health of his society. Health habits from childhood, school health activities, market hygiene, slaughter house hygiene, screening programmes, rural health check up camps etc., all help man to have the wealth of his health.

Prevention of food adulteration, Good clothing, good environmental hygiene or sanitation keeps man fit to live 100 years without illness.

Now, we know from all these things, that "**If wealth is lost something is lost, but if health is lost everything is lost.**"

My Hobby

Hobby is any type of work done for pleasure and not for gaining an earning. Hobby is the work done during our free time by which we find comfort, relaxation and joy.

Common hobbies are photography, gardening, stamp collection, coin collection, picture collection, collection of shells, painting, art, music vocal, music instrumental, mountaineering, skating, and so on.

Each one of us has his own hobbies. One person's hobby may be another person's profession. For example photography can be a hobby or an occupation or profession for earning.

My favourite hobby is photography and book writing. I am fond of drawing pictures. I collect stamps and coins whenever I get chance to get them. Thus I have collected more than 5000 stamps and more than 2000 coins. Pictures draw our attention and that is how I got into the habit of photography.

In my childhood days, in pre-independence era, camera was not easily available. One old camera called Agfa was given to me by my father, which needed to fill with film roll and exposure in an adventurous way. Its development was possible only in a studio where traditional film development was there. So, getting a photo usually used to take number of days.

As days passed by, I purchased a modern camera, which again was to be working with film roll and studio development.

Recently my son has purchased a digital camera, which is unique. He need not have film reel, he need not go to studio to develop his film! Just a set of computer does all jobs and any type and any number of photos are ready on the spot. What a change by the development of science and technology?

My classmate from USA keeps on sending photos of birds, animals and snakes. Recently I started sending photos to newspaper for publishing.

Hobby is a necessity for man. It overcomes the unnecessary worries and anxieties. It allows man to utilise his time only for necessary worries.

Truly, "**A hobby makes the man a complete man**".

The Newspapers

The news of human activities in this world reaches of your home through the newspapers. They carry the news to every household. The news comes from all directions and from all parts of the world. Truly news has no limits. The word NEWS can stand for four directions like **N**orth, **E**ast, **W**est and **S**outh.

In ancient times news had to be brought from a person who could have travelled a long distance on foot or on a horse back. The news of such transmission used to be changed by the time it reached another person, now; we see that the newspaper spreads the news all over the world in a few hours.

Historically, the newspaper began in the seventeenth century in England. In India, first newspaper was in Bengali which saw publication in 1820. Now, newspaper reaches every one even in remote areas because of improved transport technology.

Advantages of newspaper are giving fresh news of our local community, news of our state, news of our country, new law made by Government and public education. Politics cannot survive without newspaper. Culture and religion is spread by the newspaper. Sports and games are first events of newspaper. Business gives advertisement and gets benefited.

Recently school and college programmes are brought out by newspaper.

Our major National dailies are 'The Hindustan Times', 'The Hindu', 'Deccan Herald', 'Indian Express', 'The Times of India', 'Economic Times' etc.,

Our major local dailies are 'Sandhya Times', 'Samykta Karnataka', 'Prajavani', 'Vijaya Karnataka', 'Udayavani'.

I read both morning and evening dailies. It has become a habit next to daily food. I miss the newspaper if there is any holiday for the paper. Radio listening cannot give news as much as the newspaper gives.

Indeed, I am thankful to the morning and evening dailies which made me informed and modernised.

Thank you Mr. Newspapaer.

The Lady with the Lamp

Upbringing to be Deaconesses by training young women of good character is recorded in history of nursing which was started by a German pastor and his wife, Theodore and Frederica Fliedner. Duties of nurse included care of young children and religious visiting. Pastor's wife gave practical instructions, ethical lectures to many. One such girl was Florence Nightingale who was popularly called as THE LADY WITH THE LAMP by wounded soldiers of Crimean War. Nightingale campaigned without tiring to improve health standards and nursed every wounded soldier in the war.

Florence Nightingale was born to a rich couple William Edward and Frances Nightingale on 12th May 1820 in Italy. She in her younger days itself started finding answers to the social questions and started visiting the homes of the sick and investigating hospitals and nursing. It was a tough job for the rich girl to do the nursing, which was not a reputed one at that time.

A great opportunity of a life of preparation for task of care to soldiers came to Nightingale when she was asked the help by War Secretary Sidney Herbert. She then took a band of nurses out to the Crimea to give nursing care to soldiers. She had good education and from high social strata. She had great opposition from home for the above task. She set standards of practical nursing, hospital administration, which still serves as a model. She took charge of a small hospital at war time. In the army to be a "nurse of a reliable character" was a great challenge and Red tape obstructed her on all sides. Army doctors resented presence of a woman. Much worse, was the inability to face dreadful condition of war by women.

Her bravery in facing all constraints and nursing the sick soldiers made her an angel, another leading light and national heroine. Voluntary contributions by private soldiers to the tune of £ 9000 led her to start 'Nightingale Training School at St.Thomas Hospital, where nurses were trained.

In addition to laying the firm foundation of modern system of nurse training, Florence Nightingale was responsible for the total reorganisation of civil hospitals and military hospitals. She brought out many reform including improving sanitation and hygiene of Indian Army. Her pledge is vivid even today!

> "I solemnly pledge before God and in the presence of this assembly to pass my life in purity and to practice my profession faithfully. I will abstain from whatever is deleterious and mischievous and will not take or knowingly administer any harmful drug. I will do in all my power to maintain and elevate the standard of my profession and will hold in confidence all personal matters committed to my keeping and all my family affairs coming to my knowledge in the practice of my calling. With loyalty I will endeavour to aid the physician in his work, and devote myself to the welfare of those committed to my care."

She was bedridden for many years but campaigned without tiring. She was awarded Royal Red Cross in 1883 by Queen Victoria and the Order of Merit in 1907.

She died on 13th Aug 1910. Her buried body is still there near her parents' home, Embley Park in Hampshire; and her soul is still with all souls devoted to nursing care.

6.5. LETTER WRITING

Letter writing is an art. As occasion demands, all of us have to write letters to friends, relatives or officials. Hence, it is necessary that we should cultivate the art of writing different kinds of letters.

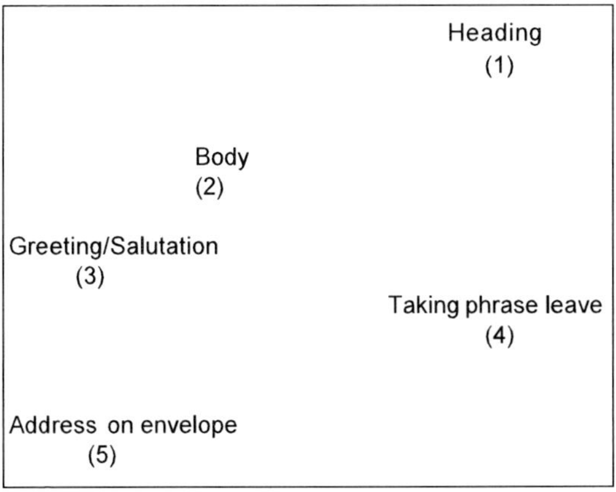

Fig 6.1: Usual format of a letter

Types of Letters

Social letters: To friend
To father
To mother
To sister
To brother

Business letters
Letters of application
Letters to newspaper

Examples of Letters

Personal:

112, Saketh Block
Sattur, Dharwad-580 008
2nd February 2006

Dear Mr.Prabhu,
It is just to wish you on your birthday and to wish you many happy returns of the day. May your future life be all bright and happy.

I didn't know what to send you for a present, but I saw an ivory idol of Ganesha the other day and bought it for you. I hope you will like it. I know your great veneration for Ganesha. We are, neither of us, as young as we used to be, and as days pass by, we are inevitably drawn to spiritual lights of Lord Ganesha.

Your old friend
Dr. GNP

Invitation:

Mrs. and Dr. (Prof) G N Prabhakara request the pleasure of the company of Mrs. and Dr. (Prof) Y S Rai at dinner on Tues, the 25th of April, 2006 at 8 O'clock.
112, Saketh Block
Sattur, Dharwad-580 009
24th April 2006

Business:

112, Saketh Block
Sattur, Dharwad-580 009
8th July 2006

Mr. Pawaninder P Vij,
M/S Peepee Publishers and Distributors (P) Ltd.,
7/31, Ansari Road, Daryaganj, P O Box 7243
New Delhi-110 002

Dear Sir,
I shall be obliged if you will send me the following books by V.P.P. at the earliest:

1. Textbook of Community Health for Nurses by Dr.G.N.Prabhakara 40 copies
2. Sociology for Nurses by Dr. G. N.Prabhakara 50 copies
3. Illustrated Nurses Dictionary by Dr.G.N.Prabhakara 100 copies
4. General Medical Dictionary by Dr.G.N.Prabhakara 50 copies
5. English for Nurses by Dr.G.N.Prabhakara and Mrs. Malathi Prabhakara 100 copies
6. Issues, Trends and Management in Nursing by Dr.G.N.Prabhakara 50 copies

Yours faithfully,
Dr. G.N.P.

Application: For Leave

7, Nurses Hostel
F N Nursing College
Kolkota
17th Sept 2006

To
The Principal
F N Nursing College
Kolkota

Respected Madam,
As I am laid up with fever since last evening, I am unable to attend the school nursing. I shall be grateful, therefore, if you will kindly grant me leave of absence for two days.

Yours obediently,
Rita H
III year student

Application: For Job

Hema Sood
112/2, Thambu Chetty Veedi
George Town, Chennai
22nd June 2006

To
The Secretary
S D M Education Society
Sattur, Dharwad-580009

Dear Sir,
In response to your advertisement in Deccan Herald for the post of Principal in Nursing College, I wish to offer myself as a candidate.

I hold M.Sc., Nursing in first lass from CMC Vellore and have 3 years of experience as Principal and am familiar with all aspects of work as Principal of a nursing college.

I enclose copies of testimonials and certificates, a certificate from my present employer the Dean, CMC Vellore.

Assuring you of my devoted services, if appointed to the post.

I remain
Yours faithfully,
Hema Sood

Official Letter:

To
The Station Director
A.I.R.
Dharwad-580 001

Sir,
As a campaign against open field defecation, we are giving health education on environmental hygiene to the community. In this connection I had written a letter to give an opportunity for four speakers to speak on different topics on the above issue.

Contd.

Contd.

Today I am sending one of my colleagues to discuss with you to plan out the AIR youth programme that can be arranged in 4 different sessions of 10 minutes each to convey the message of health hazard due to open field defecation and how to prevent it.

Please send required information for our doctors to give radio talk in your AIR scientific 'your health' programme.

Yours sincerely
Dr. GNP
Associate Dean

Letter to Newspaper:

To
The Editor
The Hindu
Mount Road, Chennai 2

Sir,

Through the columns of your esteemed daily, may I draw the attention of the Commissioner of Hubli Dharwad Municipal Corporation to the fact that some of the milk bottles distributed through the milk booths appear to have been tampered with and the milk diluted.

Of late it has been noticed that the seals of some of the bottles are loose, and the milk in such bottles is invariably found to be diluted. Milk in sealed bottle is good. Will the Commissioner of HDMC Hubli Dharwad, please, find out who is responsible for tampering with the seals and diluting the milk?

I hope that at least in future we shall be supplied with good, wholesome milk.

Yours truly
Dr.GNP

112, Saketh Block,
Sattur, Dharwad-580 009
6th April 2006

6.6. NURSES' NOTES

Nurse takes the every round with doctor and takes the instructions in the rounds. Her routine rounds cover the following areas:

Ward rounds
OT notes
Surgical case notes
Out patient notes
Investigation notes
Post operative notes
Child guidance notes
Immunisation notes

Examples of Nurses Notes:

Instructions for OT case:

8th Sept morning rounds
evening Nembutal pre medication
9th morning 6 AM another dose Nembutal
early morning urine specimen collect and send for examination
No fluid after 7 AM
Prepare with OT dress, hair brushed, covered with a cap, jewellery removed
7.30 AM catheterise
7.45 AM atropine, anaesthetic check up

Instructions in ward rounds:

Case Anal fissure
Prepare for anal dilatation (one finger)
Prepare for soap enema

Case preoperative GJ
Prepare for gastric aspiration and send for diagnostic purpose

Case Ulcer foot
Dress and bandage
Continue antibiotic

Case: Enteric fever
Arrange for Widal test
Prepare temp. chart, pulse chart and BP chart 4th hrly
Continue paracetemol as suggested

6.7. HEALTH PROBLEM REPORTS

Nurse has to interact with patients in different disciplines. Accordingly health problem report making is utmost important in day-to-day nursing care services.

Day care and night duty care needs observation and a report has to be prepared including the nursing care given.

Health problem report has to be submitted to tutor, matron, nursing superintendent and to the attending doctor for their advice and instructions for continued care.

Examples of health problem reports:

Case head injury concussion.

Hourly pulse, respiration and BP recorded and entered in the chart.

Nausea is preceded by retching; it is accompanied by pain. The material is saved for inspection and note is made of the quantity of the vomit and the number of times of vomiting in 24 hours.

Drugs given as per the instructions.

Patient had one attack of convulsion. Duty doctor was called who gave parenteral medication.

Pulse, Respiratory rate and BP were checked.
IV line secured.
Assessed for the need for IV fluids/osmolar agents (based on clinical status).
Patient is not sedated even though he is not cooperating, as per the instructions.
Prepared and shifted the case for CT scan.

After the return of patient, Assessed the vitals and the need for IV fluids based on the BP. Patient is started with IV fluid.

Case is handed over with the report to the right duty nurse at 8 PM.

6.8. RESUME OR CURRICULUM VITAE

Along with an application, one has to apply for a suitable job that requires summary of the academic accumulations.

It is preferred to give vital information on academic achievement and experience so that it will be useful for the committee for selection to assess the candidate.

This is also called as Bio Data of the candidate. Usual format includes some identification data, date of birth, qualification, additional qualification, extra curricular activities, experience in the field.

Name:	Ms. Shakuntala
Age:	21 years
Date of birth:	2.10.84
Father's name:	A G Narasimha
Residential address:	25, T K layout, SWT Koppal 4th stage, Saraswathipuram Mysore 570 009
Contact number:	0821-2544436
Qualification:	B.Sc., Nursing First Class M.Sc., Nursing First Class 2 months special training in OT Nursing
Teaching experience:	Nil
Experience:	Worked as OT Nurse in CMC Vellore for 6 months
Extra Curricular Activities:	Inter-university chess champion Represented nursing college in Debate

Chapter 7 Vocabulary

7.1. ANTONYM

Antonyms are words of the same grammatical class such as nouns, verbs or adjectives that have opposite meanings.

Words	*Antonyms*
Attract	Repel
Awake	Asleep
Above	Beneath, below
Abstract	Concrete
Accept	Reject
Acquit	Condemn
Advance	Retreat
Affirm	Deny
Affluence	Poverty
Aggravate	Alleviate, lessen
Agree	Differ
Allow	Forbid
Analysis	Synthesis
Ancient	Modern
Arrive	Depart
Asset	Liability
Ability	Disability
Abundance	Dearth
Accord	Discord
Admire	Dislike
Adopt	Reject
Appreciate	Depreciate
Arrival	Departure
Arrogant	Humble
Artificial	Natural
Attack	Defend
Attract	Repel

Awkward	Graceful
Normal	Abnormal
Accelerate	Slowness
Belief	Doubt
Barren	Fertile
Bold	Timid
Bona fide	Mala fides
Bravery	Cowardice
Bright	Dull, dim
Centrifugal	Centripetal
Cheap	Costly
Cheerful	Gloomy
Clean	Dirty
Clever	Stupid
Common	Rare
Compulsory	Optional
Confident	Uncertain
Convex	Concave
Create	Destroy
Barbarous	Civilised
Bliss	Misery
Borrow	Lend
Brutal	Humane
Callous	Sensitive
Care	Neglect
Cautious	Rash
Certain	Uncertain
Coarse	Fine
Comic	Tragic
Compare	Contrast
Competent	Incompetent
Compress	Expand
Conceal	Reveal
Condense	Expand
Continue	Discontinue
Costly	Cheap
Credit	Debit
Crude	Refined
Cruel	Kind
Darkness	Brightness
Danger	Safety
Dawn	Dusk
Debit	Credit
Deduction	Induction
Deep	Shallow
Defendant	Plaintiff

Defensive	Offensive
Deficit	Surplus
Deflate	Inflate
Deliberate	Unintentional
Democracy	Autocracy
Diligent	Lazy
Dilute	Concentrated
Dwarf	Giant
Decrease	Increase
Definite	Indefinite
Delay	Haste
Delight	Displeasure, sorrow
Dense	Sparse
Descend	Ascend
Destruction	Construction
Diffident	Confident
Discourage	Encourage
Distant	Near
Egoism	Altruism
Elevation	Depression
Emigrant	Immigrant
Exaggeration	Understatement
Exclude	Include
Exit	Entrance
Exotic	Indigenous
Expand	Contract
Explicit	Implicit
Exterior	Interior
External	Internal
Extravagant	Thrifty
Early	Late
Earthly	Heavenly
Economy	Extravagance
Eligible	Ineligible
End	Beginning
Energetic	Weal
Enmity	Friendship
Equality	Inequality
Enthusiasm	Indifference
Exceptional	Ordinary
Experience	Inxperience
Famous	Obscure
Fast	Slow, loose
Fat	Thin, lean
Flattery	Detraction
Float	Sink

Foreign	Native
Forget	Remember
Frequent	Rare
Fresh	Stale
Friendly	Hostile
Full	Empty
Fabulous	Real, actual
Fact	Fiction
Failure	Success
Fair	Foul
False	True
Familiar	Strange
Fanciful	Practical
Ferocious	Mild, gentle
Fickle	Constant
Fictitious	True, genuine
Fine	Coarse
Flexible	Rigid, stiff
Freedom	Slavery
Futility	Utility
Gain	Loss
Gather	Scatter
General	Particular, special
Generous	Mean
Gentle	Rough
Genuine	Spurious
Gradual	Sudden, abrupt
Grave	Gay
Guilty	Innocent
Harsh	Gentle
Hasty	Leisurely
Hate	Love
Heavy	Light
Help	Hinder
Hero	Villain
High	Low
Hit	Miss
Hollow	Solid
Homogeneous	Heterogeneous
Honour	Shame
Hope	Despair
Host	Guest
Hurt	Heal
Gaiety	Mourning
Gain	Loss
Gloomy	Gay

Good	Bad
Growth	Decline
Happiness	Sorrow, sadness
Hard	Soft
Honest	Dishonest
Humane	Cruel
Humble	Proud
Humility	Arrogance
Hypocrisy	Sincerity
Ideal	Actual
Idle	Busy
Imagination	Reality
Import	Export
Increase	Decrease
Individual	General
Industrious	Lazy, indolent
Inferior	Superior
Inhale	Exhale
Input	Output
Insert	Extract
Imperative	Optional
Include	Exclude
Interested	Disinterested
Interesting	Uninteresting
Jovial	Gloomy, morose
Joy	Sorrow
Junior	Senior
Justify	Condemn
Justice	Injustice
Keen	Dull, blunt
Kill	Resurrect
Kind	Cruel
Kindle	Extinguish
King	Subject
Knowledge	Ignorance
Landlord	Tenant
Later	Earlier
Latitude	Longitude
Lead	Follow
Lend	Borrow
Literal	Figurative
Loose	Tight
Lack	Plenty
Legal	Illegal
Legible	Illegible
Liberty	Slavery

Light	Heavy
Liquid	Solid
Long	Short
Love	Hate
Loyal	Treacherous
Major	Minor
Many	Few
Marriage	Celibacy
Masculine	Feminine
Material	Spiritual
Maximum	Minimum
Memory	Oblivion
Micro	Macro
Mild	Severe
Miser	Spendthrift
Monogamy	Polygamy
Monotony	Variety, diversity
Motion	Rest
Mad	Sane
Malice	Goodwill
Master	Servant
Meagre	Plentiful
Melancholy	Gaiety
Merit	Demerit
Mighty	Weak
Miserly	Stern, harsh
Moral	Immoral
Morbid	Healthy
Mortal	Immortal
Narrow	Broad
Native	Foreign
Natural	Artificial
Nebulous	Distinct, clear
Negative	Positive
Neutral	Partial
Niggard	Spendthrift
Noxious	Wholesome
Neat	Untidy
Noble	Ignoble
Normal	Abnormal
Notorious	Reputable
Observe	Reverse
Odd	Even
Offer	Refuse
Often	Seldom
Omission	Commission

Optimistic	Pessimistic
Oral	Written
Oriental	Occidental
Original	Duplicate, copy
Orthodox	Heterodox
Ostensible	Actual
Partly	Wholly
Permanent	Temporary
Permit	Prohibit
Philanthropist	Misanthropist
Pleasure	Pain
Practice	Theory
Pragmatic	Idealistic
Praise	Blame
Precede	Succeed
Pride	Humility
Profit	Loss
Progress	Regress
Progressive	Retrograde
Promote	Demote
Prow	Stern
Public	Private
Part	Whole
Partial	Impartial, fair
Particular	General
Passion	Coolness
Pathetic	Joyous
Peace	War
Persuade	Dissuade
Physical	Mental, spiritual
Please	Displease
Plenty	Scarcity
Polite	Rude, impolite
Poor	Rich, wealthy
Practicable	Impracticable
Precious	Cheap, worthless
Premium	Discount
Prospect	Retrospect
Prosperity	Adversity
Prudent	Imprudent
Punishment	Reward
Pure	Impure
Quiet	Noisy
Queer	Normal
Quarrelsome	Friendly, peaceful
Quick	Slow, tardy

Rash	Careful, cautious
Rapid	Slow, leisurely
Recede	Advance
Relative	Absolute
Reluctant	Willing, ready
Remember	Forget
Remitter	Receiver, recipient
Reserved	Sociable
Resist	Submit
Retail	Wholesale
Reward	Punish
Rigid	Flexible
Ripe	Raw
Rise	Fall, set
Rough	Smooth
Rude	Polite
Raise	Lower
Rare	Ordinary, common
Rash	Cautious, steady
Real	False
Rear	Front
Receive	Give
Rectify	Falsify
Reject	Accept, admit
Relevant	Irrelevant
Religious	Secular, irreligious
Relish	Dislike
Remote	Near
Repulsive	Attractive
Rich	Poor, needy
Right	Wrong
Sacred	Secular
Safe	Dangerous
Saint	Sinner
Servant	Master
Sharp	Blunt
Simple	Complex
Sink	Float
Smile	Frown
Sober	Rash
Solid	Liquid
Straight	Curved
Strait	Broad
Strange	Familiar
Subjective	Objective
Succeed	Fail

Sure	Doubtful
Sweet	Bitter
Sympathy	Antipathy
Sane	Insane
Satisfaction	Dissatisfaction
Savage	Civilised
Scanty	Plentiful
Secret	Public, open
Sensible	Insensible, senseless
Sensitive	Insensitive
Separate	Joint
Service	Disservice
Severe	Mild
Shy	Bold, impudent
Silence	Noise
Sin	Virtue
Smart	Dull, slow
Soft	Hard, stubborn
Sophisticated	Naïve
Sorrow	Joy
Special	Ordinary
Speedy	Slow
Spiritual	Material
Stale	Fresh
Stationary	Moving
Sublime	Ridiculous
Success	Failure
Sufficient	Insufficient
Superior	Inferior
Surplus	Deficit
Swift	Slow
Synonym	Antonym
Tall	Short
Temporal	Eternal
Tense	Relaxed
Terrestrial	Celestial
Thesis	Antithesis
Thick	Thin
Tight	Loose
Top	Bottom
Tranquil	Agitated
Transparent	Opaque
Triumph	Defeat
Trivial	Important
True	False
Tame	Wild

Tedious	Lively
Tender	Hard, strong
Thankful	Thankless
Theory	Practice
Thin	Thick, fat, stout
Thrive	Decline
Timid	Bold
Tolerance	Intolerance
Tragic	Comic
Transient	Lasting, durable
Unite	Separate
Upper	Lower
Upright	Dishonest
Urban	Rural
Ugly	Rude
Uniform	Variable
Union	Disunion
Use	Disuse
Useful	Useless
Usual	Unusual
Vacant	Occupied
Vague	Clear
Variable	Constant
Vanguard	Rearguard
Vertical	Horizontal
Victory	Defeat
Virtue	Vice
Voluntary	Involuntary
Vain	Modest
Vigilant	Careless, heedless
Vindictive	Forgiving
Violent	Gentle
Visible	Invisible
Vulgar	Refined
Wake	Sleep
Wax	Wane
Wealth	Poverty
Wide	Narrow
Win	Lose
Wise	Foolish
Wane	Wax
Want	Abundance
War	Peace
Warmth	Coolness
Wearisome	Refreshing
Weighty	Light

Wild	Civilised
Woeful	Cheerful
Work	Idleness
Wrong	Right
Yield	Resist
Youth	Age
Zenith	Nadir
Zeal	Indifference

7.2. SYNONYM

They are words of the same grammatical class that have similar meaning. It is not exactly the same meaning but is similar meaning. Here the words convey same general notion. Take the examples of following words:

Kill	*She was killed.*
Murder	*He was murdered.*
Slaughter	*Sheep was slaughtered.*
Slay	*Captain was slain in the battle.*
Execute	*Criminal was executed.*

Though they are used in different contexts and in different senses they are treated as synonyms.

Words	*Synonyms*
Abbreviate	Abridge, condense, shorten, curtail, prune
Abdomen	Belly, paunch, epigastrium
Abnormal	Aberrant, irregular, anomalous
Abortion	Miscarriage, premature delivery
Accelerate	Hasten, expedite, speed up, quicken
Accident	Mishap, injury, casualty
Addict	Devotee, fan, habitual user, slave to
Admission	Concession, confession, entry, admittance
Adolescence	Youth, teens, puberty
Affect	Influence, concern
Agony	Pain, torture, anguish
Amnesia	Forgetfulness, loss of memory
Anaemia	Bloodlessness, lack of blood
Anatomy	Body structure, framework, zootomy
Approach	Nearing, advent, coming, approximation
Attenuate	Weaken, thin out, rarefy
Autopsy	Post mortem, cadaver examination
Accomplish	Achieve, perform
Adversity	Calamity, misfortune
Amusement	Diversion, recreation

Anger	Ire, wrath, rage
Aversion abduct	Dislike, antipathy
Accede	Consent, agree
Adoration	Worship, love
Aggravate	Intensify, heighten
Apprehend	Fear, perceive
Attack	Aggression, invasion, assault
Audacious	Daring, bold
Awkward	Clumsy, odd
Baby	Infant, child, offspring
Bed	Couch, cot, resting place
Benefit	Profit, advantage, gain, avail
Bland	Affable, mild, unflavoured, gracious
Blanket	Covering, conceal
Bleed	Flow, haemorrhage, overcharge, suffer
Bloodletting	Phlebotomy, venesection
Body	Anatomy, structure, form
Boil	Sore, suppuration
Bony	Skeletal, stiff, osseous
Breath	Respiration, inhalation, breeze
Breast	Bosom, bust, mamma
Breed	Create, multiply, generate, produce
Buttocks	Rump, seat, breech
Blend	Mix, mingle
Bondage	Slavery
Brave	Courageous, bold
Brief	Concise, short
Beautiful	Attractive, lovely, charming
Behaviour	Demeanour, manner
Blunder	Big mistake
Build	Construct
Callous	Horny, tough, hardened
Castrate	Emasculate, unman, geld
Casualty	Chance, accident, disaster, calamity
Cathartic	Laxative, purgative, aperients
Cavity	Hole, excavation, hollow, pit
Cell	Protoplasm, cage, compartment
Census	Poll, count, enumeration
Chest	Case, box, cabinet, breast
Child	Tot, son, daughter
Christmas	Yule, Noel
Chronic	Persistent, continuing, constant
Closet	Cabinet, wardrobe, cubby-hole
Community	Neighbourhood, society, group
Compassion	Sympathy, kindness, mercy
Component	Integral part, element, constituent

Conceive	Frame, become pregnant, grasp
Condition	Fitness, state, rank
Consanguinity	Kin, relationship, blood tie
Consent	Assent, agreement, compliance
Contact	Touch, connection, liaison
Contagion	Communicability, infection
Coordinate	Equalise, adapt, adjust
Cordial	Sincere, hearty, tie
Correlation	Reciprocal ness, mutuality
Couple	Join, link, marry, link
Culture	Development, breeding, cultivation
Cure	Heal, relieve, preserve
Cycle	Period, circle, round
Check	Restrain, stop, curb
Compel	Coerce, force
Confuse	Confound, perplex
Callous	Cruel, ruthless
Corrupt	Tainted, debased
Compassion	Pity, sympathy
Dead	Deceased, perished, lifeless
Deaf	Hard of hearing, unhearing
Delinquent	Neglectful, culpable, defaulting
Demonstration	Substantiation, exhibition, display
Differentiate	Neglectful, culpable, defaulting
Discharge	Dismiss, retire, fire, pay
Discrimination	Differentiation, distinction
Disinfect	Sterilise, purify, cleanse
Dislocate	Displace, disjoin, disarrange
Displacement	Dispossession, removal, ousting
Distend	Stretch, expand, dilate, swell
Doctor	Physician, surgeon, learned man
Domestic	Household, homely, family, tame
Donation	Contribution, gift, present, grant
Drain	Draw off, empty, exhaust, deprive
Drip	Drop, dribble, trickle, percolate
Dull	Unsharp, blunt, stupid, slow
Dwarf	Midget, pygmy, Lilliputian
Degeneration	Deterioration
Deplorable	Regrettable, lamentable
Divide	Part, separate
Damage	Harm, loss, injury
Danger	Stake, hazard, peril
Deadly	Fatal, lethal
Decay	Fade, wither, spoil
Decorate	Adorn, embellish
Deficient	Wanting, lacking

Deformity	Defect, malformation
Delicious	Dainty, exquisite
Delicate	Brittle, soft
Destitute	Wanting, needy
Disseminate	Spread, scatter
Dread	Fear, horror
Ear	Auricle, concha, hearing sense organ
Ego	Self, personality
Eliminate	Expel, remove, exclude
Eradicate	Abolish, erase, exterminate
Eruption	Rash, discharge, outbreak
Example	Sample, specimen, piece
Excitability	Violence, passion, rage
Exhale	Breathe, expel, emit, respire
Exude	Emit, discharge, leak
Eccentric	Peculiar, odd
Efficient	Able, competent
Endure	Suffer, tolerate
Enormous	Huge, immense
Error	Mistake, blunder
Eternal	Timeless, perpetual
Eager	Anxious, enthusiastic
Eccentric	Odd, singular
Emulate	Follow, imitate
Extravagant	Lavish, wasteful, spendthrift
Face	Features, front, countenance
Faint	Lose heart, fail, weaken
Fatigue	Tire, exhaust, bore
Feed	Eat, dine, graze, furnish
Fluid	Liquid, juice, blood, solution
Fracture	Break, split, crack, cleft
Famous	Renowned, celebrated
Feeble	Weak, infirm
Ferocious	Fierce, savage
Foolish	Silly, stupid
Frank	Candid, open
False	Untrue, spurious
Fecund	Fertile, productive
Feminine	Female, womanly, womanish
Fiction	Myth, fabrication
Fraud	Trickery, deceit
Fury	Wrath, anger
Germ	Micro organism, seed, embryo
Gigantic	Monstrous, elephantine, titanic, huge
Grain	Fruit, cereal, seed, kernel
Gymnastics	Athletics, exercises, acrobatics

General	Universal
Gentle	Tender, mild, kind
Giggle	Laugh, titter
Grave	Sober, serious
Grief	Sorrow, pain, agony
Guard	Defend, protect
Gaiety	Happiness, hilarity
Genuine	Real
Gorgeous	Splendid, dazzling
Gratification	Satisfaction, enjoyment
Grief	Pain, sorrow, regret
Guilt	Crime, sin
Hair	Filament, bristles, pile
Hallucination	Phantasm, phantom, mirage, delusion
Hazard	Danger, chance, risk, accident
Helmet	Headgear, skullcap, headpiece
Hereditary	Inheritable, transmissible, ancestral
Hospital	Sanatorium, clinic, infirmary
Hospitality	Sociality, cordiality, welcome
Host	Mass, element, throng, multitude
Human	Mortal, humane, civilised
Hurt	Damage, pain, ache, wound, loss
Hybrid	Mixture, crossbreed, cross
Hypnotic	Mesmeric, fascinating, narcotic
Hypothesis	Supposition, theory, postulate, assumption
Hysterical	Uncontrolled, wild, emotional
Habit	Custom, practice
Hinder	Obstruct, prevent
Holy	Sacred
Hamper	Hinder, retard, impede
Harmony	Uniformity, union, consent
Humility	Modesty, humbleness
Idiocy	Imbecility, cretinism, feeblemindedness
Ill	Unwell, sick, nauseous
Improvement	Uplift, betterment, advancement
Impulse	Impetus, momentum, push, thrust
Incident	Occasion, event, episode, happening
Incompatible	Inconsistent, inharmonious, clashing
Indication	Denotation, signification, symbolism
Infancy	Babyhood, childhood, cradle, genesis
Infant	Baby, babe, child, offspring
Infection	Contagion, illness, epidemic
Inheritance	Bequest, legacy, patrimony
Insect	Bug, fly, moth, beetle
Insertion	Inlay, introduction, impregnation
Insomnia	Sleeplessness, wakefulness

Intercourse	Communication, coitus, congress
Intern	Confine, detain, student doctor
Investigate	Inquire, examine, question, search
Isolation	Separation, quarantine, segregation
Itch	Desire to scratch, tickling, prickly sense
Idle	Lazy, indolent
Illegal	Unlawful, lawless
Include	Comprise
Increase	Enlarge, augment
Irritation	Annoyance, vexation
Illiterate	Ignorant, unlearned
Impertinent	Shameless, insolent
Impostor	Cheat
Ingenious	Clever, inventive
Intend	Propose, mean
Jerk	Twist, pull, tweak
Juvenile	Youngster, minor, adolescent
Jealous	Envious
Just	Fair, impartial
Jubilant	Happy, joyful
Keen	Sharp
Kind	Benevolent
King	Monarch, ruler
Knowledge	Recognition, information
Labyrinth	Complexity, intricacy, maze
Lame	Crippled, ineffectual, weak
Latency	Passivity, dormancy, silence
Lateral	Sidelong
Legitimate	Lawful, legal, genuine
Limb	Arm, leg, branch, member
Lucid	Clear, transparent, rational
Lump	Protuberance, swelling, mass
Lens	Eyeglass, reading glass, refractor
Lethargy	Lassitude, apathy, stupor
Labour	Work, toil
Latent	Dormant, hidden
Learning	Knowledge, scholarship
Liberal	Generous
Lie	Falsehood
Loyal	True, faithful
Laborious	Diligent, hardworking
Liberty	Freedom, independence
Lucky	Fortunate
Luxuriant	Abundant, profuse
Machine	Apparatus, device, engine
Mad	Crazy, insane, rabid, turbulent

Malady	Disease, sickness, infirmity
Malformation	Distortion, deformity
Malpractice	Improper treatment, misconduct
Mania	Madness, lunacy, insanity
Maturity	Ripeness, adulthood
Medicine	Remedy , drugs, therapy
Melancholy	Dejected, sad, depressed
Mild	Gentle, easy, harmless
Mouth	Entrance, oral cavity, lips
Muscular	Strong, brawny, vigorous
Myth	Legend, tradition, fiction
Magnificent	Splendid, stately
Malady	Illness, disease
Miserly	Stingy, closefisted
Modest	Unassuming, bashful
Mourn	Lament
Malice	Ill will, spite
Meagre	Small, low
Merciful	Pitiful, compassionate
Mockery	Ridicule, derision
Nail	Ungula, claw, fingernail
Naked	Uncovered, bare, stripped, unclothed
Nausea	Seasickness, aversion, illness
Nearsighted	Short-sighted, myopic
Nourishment	Food, sustenance, nutrient
Nuptial	Bridal, connubial, wed
Nurse	Nursemaid, attendant, nanny, foster
Negligent	Careless, heedless
Nice	Pleasant, agreeable
Notable	Memorable, remarkable
Notorious	Infamous
Nasty	Filthy, dirty
Nativity	Birth
Need	Necessity
Noble	Illustrious, lofty
Norm	Standard
Novice	Beginner
Oath	Curse, epithet, pledge, bond
Obese	Overweight, plump, fleshy, bulky
Occupation	Tenure, holding, work, trade, business
Occurrence	Event, happening, episode, phenomenon
Optimism	Hopefulness, encouragement, enthusiasm
Optional	Voluntary, discretionary, elective
Oral	Verbal, vocal, spoken, unwritten
Oval	Elliptical, ovoid, ovate
Ovum	Cell, egg, seed

Obscene	Filthy, indecent
Obstacle	Hindrance
Obvious	Clear, evident
Odd	Strange, peculiar
Ornament	Adornment, jewel
Obliterate	Destroy, efface
Obtuse	Dull, stupid
Ostentation	Sow, display
Pale	Ashy, colourless, bloodless
Pallor	Paleness, wanness, colourlessness
Panacea	Universal remedy, cure-all
Parasite	Sycophant, leech, bloodsucker,
Parental	Motherly, fatherly, protective, loving
Penetrate	Bore, burrow, pierce, enter
Perennial	Lasting, enduring, endless, persistent
Perform	Enact, play, execute, fulfil
Pernicious	Malign, poisonous, detrimental
Pervert	Distort, twist
Pest	Plague, parasite, trouble, curse
Pharmacist	Chemist, apothecary, druggist
Phonetic	Sonant, voiced, lingual
Physician	Doctor, surgeon, healer, consultant
Pierce	Puncture, penetrate, perforate
Placard	Notice, poster, billboard
Plastic	Mouldable, malleable, impressionable
Pledge	Promise, security, pan, collateral
Plump	Chubby, stout, fleshy
Poignant	Painful, pungent, intense
Poisonous	Venomous, toxic, deadly
Pollute	Contaminate, foul, soil, corrupt
Population	Inhabitants, people, residents
Position	Situation, placement, spot
Practical	Pragmatical, useful, operative, effective
Pray	Implore, ask, beg
Precaution	Care, warning, safeguard
Prescribe	Urge, suggest, order, advocate
Prevalence	Dominance, ubiquitousness
Prevention	Hindrance, preclusion, inhibition
Primary	Chief, original, initial, first
Privacy	Seclusion, solitude, secrecy
Probation	Trial, test, examination
Problem	Question, proposition, exercise, puzzle
Profession	Vocation, calling, occupation
Prominent	Notable, important, salient, memorable
Pronunciation	Utterance, saying, voicing, articulation
Propaganda	Publicity, persuasion, movement

Prophylactic	Preventive, precautionary, protective
Proportion	Dimension, ratio, share, part
Protuberance	Projection, bulge, prominence, swelling
Pseudo	Spurious, counterfeit, simulated
Puncture	Perforation, hole, opening
Pupil	Student, schoolchild, learner
Pus	Matter, suppuration, purulence
Pardon	Forgive, excuse
Permit	Allow
Precise	Exact
Premature	Hasty
Proficient	Adept, expert
Profuse	Lavish, extravagant
Project	Plan, scheme
Proprietor	Owner
Proverb	Saw, adage
Prudent	Discreet, wise, sagacious
Pain	Ache, agony, anguish
Pathetic	Moving, touching
Perennial	Perpetual, permanent
Pious	Holy, sacred, devout
Plentiful	Ample, abundant
Precarious	Risky, dangerous, hazardous
Quake	Shake
Quantum	Amount, share
Queer	Strange, eccentric
Quest	Search
Quit	Leave, depart
Quiver	Tremble, shiver
Questionable	Doubtful
Radical	Fundamental, drastic, sweeping
Rapid	Swift, speedy, fleet
Ratification	Confirmation, validation, approval
Reaction	Response, reflex, revulsion
Receipt	Reception, income proceeds
Recognition	Identification, perception, cognisance
Recom-mendation	Testimonial, suggestion, advocacy
Recovery	Restitution, retrieval, reclamation
Recurrence	Repetition, return, periodicity
Reduce	Diminish, lessen, curtail
Reference	Citation, testimonial, credentials
Rejection	Exclusion, repudiation
Relapse	Recurrence, deterioration, regression
Remission	Cancellation, annulment, suspension
Repair	Restore, remedy

Requirement	Want, necessity, requisite
Resignation	Retirement, renunciation, quitting
Resonance	Vibration, resounding, rebound
Restless	Nervous, impatient, disturbed
Resuscitate	Revive, restore, reanimate
Retardation	Delay, slow down, hindrance
Rubbish	Waste, debris, litter, junk
Rupture	Split, falling-out, discord
Rare	Scarce, infrequent
Recover	Regain, retrieve
Relate	Tell, narrate
Remember	Recollect, recall
Reserved	Reticent
Residue	Remainder, remnant
Respect	Esteem, regard
Restraint	Restriction, curb
Revenge	Vengeance, retribution
Reverence	Veneration
Rude	Impolite, discourteous
Radiant	Bright, brilliant
Refined	Civilised, elegant
Rejoice	Delight
Relevant	Pertinent
Remote	Far, distant
Resistance	Opposition
Ridiculous	Absurd, laughable
Rigid	Stiff, stern
Ruin	Downfall, destruct
Savage	Cruel, barbarous
Scold	Rebuke, reprimand, censure
Secret	Hidden
Sense	Meaning, import
Severe	Strict, stern
Shy	Coy, bashful
Solitary	Lonely
Superfluous	Unnecessary, needless
Sympathy	Compassion, fellow feeling
Sacred	Holy, pious
Sane	Sound, sensible
Scandal	Slander, infamy
Scanty	Meagre, less
Serious	Grave, solemn
Simple	Plain, natural
Solace	Relief, comfort
Solitary	Single, lonely
Sordid	Dirty, ugly

Special	Distinctive, particular
Specimen	Sample, model
Spurious	False, fictitious
Static	Fixed
Sterile	Unproductive, barren
Sublime	Elevate, exalted
Submission	Surrender, obedience
Superficial	Shallow, unwanted
Synonymous	Equivalent, similar
Salary	Stipend, pay, remuneration
Screen	Partition, curtain, shield, mask
Secretary	Clerk, administrator,
Serious	Grave, earnest, important
Service	Aid, help, duty, employment
Session	Sitting, meeting, semester, hearing
Sex	Gender, sexuality, male, female
Shake	Vibrate, agitate, shiver, rock
Shave	Graze, mark down, trim
Shock	Jolt, surprise, horrify, stun
Sickly	Invalid, unwell, pale
Sight	Vision, eyesight view, scene
Signify	Show, declare, denote, indicate
Skeleton	Frame, outline, bones, diagram
Skin	Peel, cuticle, dermis
Sleep	Somnolence, nap, doze
Slim	Slender, thin, weak
Small	Little, short, minute
Soap	Cleanser, lather, detergent, shampoo
Society	Fold, culture, group, mankind
Solvent	Moneyed, financially sound, responsible
Sorry	Regretful, pitiful, sorrowful
Specialise	Concentrate on one thing, work in one field, be specific
Sperm	Semen, seed, germ
Spinster	Maid, maiden, old maid
Spontaneous	Instinctive, automatic
Stable	Stall, barn
Steward	Trustee, provider, caterer
Stigma	Brand, blemish, birthmark
Stimulate	Excite, rouse, animate
Stipend	Compensation, wage, pay
Stomach	Hunger, appetite, belly
Stool	Seat, cricket, hassock
Subject	Topic, theme, citizen
Sudden	Abrupt, unexpected, quick
Suffer	Sustain, tolerate, endure, undergo

Suicide	Self destruction, self ruin
Supernatural	Miraculous, unearthly, superhuman
Survey	View, inspect, appraise
Suspect	Infer, imagine, surmise
Sustain	Bear up, maintain, prolong
Swallow	Ingest, gulp, devour, consume
Swell	Expand, bulge, protrude
Symmetry	Shapeliness, beauty, proportion
Sympathy	Agreement, understanding, accord
Taboo	Forbiddance, prohibition
Tackle	Gear, equipment, address
Task	Work, job, lesson, assignment
Team	Crew, play team
Tears	Weeping, crying
Technique	Execution, method
Tender	Offer, propose, present
Tension	Strain, anxiety, nervousness
Tincture	Tint, shade, trace, touch
Tissue	Fabric, mesh, cartilage, muscle
Tobacco	Smoking, cigar, snuff
Tongue	Organ of taste, dialect, projection
Tooth	Canine, incisor, molar, fang
Tranquilise	Pacify, soothe, calm
Tremor	Shivering, shaking, vibration
Tropical	Hot, equatorial
Teach	Instruct, educate
Tedious	Tiresome
Tender	Soft, delicate
Timid	Shy, diffident
Tradition	Custom, convention
Transparent	Clear, lucid
Talkative	Garrulous
Tame	Gentle, mild
Temporal	Worldly, terrestrial
Theatrical	Dramatic
Tough	Hard, strong
Ulcer	Infection, abscess, sore
Unhealthy	Sickly, ailing, frail
Union	Connection, joining, unity
Unprepared	Unready, incomplete
Unsuccessful	Unfortunate, unprosperous
Usual	Customary, habitual, ordinary
Ubiquitous	Omnipresent
Ultimate	Final, last
Undergo	Suffer, endure
Unique	Incomparable, unequalled

Ugly	Repulsive
Unique	Matchless, unequalled
Urge	Incite, press
Vagabond	Wanderer, vagrant
Valid	Sound, legal, logical
Vein	Blood vessel, streak
Vermin	Pests, insects
Vigilant	Alert, watchful, careful
Virile	Potent, masculine
Visibility	Conspicuity, distinctness
Visit	Call, interview, stopover
Vital	Essential, necessary, life supporting
Voice	Speak, singing, intonation
Voluntary	Free-will, unasked, unforced
Vacant	Void, empty
Vacation	Holiday
Vague	Indistinct
Vulgar	Indecent, coarse
Waist	Girth, loin, middle
Weak	Feeble, powerless
Wheeze	Gasp, breathe hard
Wholesome	Beneficial, healthy
Win	Beat, conquer
Word	Syllable, expression, utterance
Wound	Injury, hurt, pain
Wrong	Injustice, erroneousness
Xanthous	Golden hair, yellowish, mongolism
X-ray	Roentgen ray, radiograph
Yawn	Gape, open wide, part
Yeast	Ferment, foam
Yield	Surrender, submit
Yearly	Annual
Zeal	Devotion, dedication
Zip	Energy, vigour
Zenith	Top, summit

7.3. ONE WORD

They are called one word substitutes for phrases and clauses. All languages have such one word to express certain concepts and definitions. So much so English too has the one word substitution.

They are developed through local dialect, local custom and local tradition. Learning one word substitutes helps in developing a good vocabulary.

Following list gives a carefully selected list of one word substitutes. Study them closely to increase your vocabulary.

When once you understand the meaning or concept, learn to use them in sentences of your own.

One word	*Their meaning*
Aborigines	The original inhabitants of a place
Accomplice	A partner in crime
Ambiguous	Interpreted in double meaning
Amphibian	Animal that lives both on land and in water
Anniversary	Yearly celebration of a vital event
Anonymous	Whose name is not known but does a job
Antibiotics	Drugs which kill pathogens or germs
Antidote	Medicine which counteracts to clear poison (from vermin bite or consumed)
Antiseptic	That which prevents sepsis or infection
Aquarium	Decorative mini tank to keep live fishes
Archaeology	Study of prehistoric events including antiquities
Architect	Engineer who designs and decorates the buildings
Artist	A professional dancer, musician, singer
Astronaut	Person who travels in spaceship in the orbit
Atheism	No belief or what so ever in the existence of God
Audience	Gathering gathered for a show
Autobiography	Life study written by a person on himself
Autocrat	Ruler with absolute power not subject to any control
Aviation	Understanding the design and flying of aircrafts
Anarchy	No ruler for a nation or no government
Autocracy	One ruler ruling the nation with command
Accelerate	Increase the rate or speed of an act
Adolescence	The period of growth between childhood and adulthood
Assimilate	To digest and absorb completely
Aggravate	Increase in severity or intensity
Amateur	Non professional, novice
Auditor	Person who does accounting and fiscal examination
Barricade	Barrier erected temporarily in a place
Boycott	Outcasting from all social, spiritual and commercial relations

Bureaucracy	Government run by bureaucrats who are called government servants
Bigot	Person who is prejudiced with religion
Blaspheme	Impious talk on scared things
Botany	Scientific study of plant kingdom
Biology	Scientific study of plant and animal kingdom (both zoology and botany)
Cannibal	One who eats human flesh
Capitalism	Dominated by industrialists and business-men
Carnivorous	Animals which eat flesh of other animals
Cartoon	Humorous illustrations with funny pictures
Coexistence	To live together with harmony
Colleague	Professional or official associate
Collusion	To deceive others, two parties have some secret understandings
Complacent	The satisfaction obtained by one's own achievement
Compromise	Disputes or differences are settled
Computer	Electronic device to compute, store and analyse material and data
Consensus	All parties coming to an agreement on an issue
Contemporary	People living in the same century
Cosmopolitan	A place where people can live without pre-judice and with universal brotherhood
Credulous	Innocent who believes everything
Callous	Hard hearted or without sympathy
Consummation	To become pregnant, to bring an act into completion
Congenital	Defect present since birth
Collaborator	Person who has joined in the effort of another person
Deadlock	Progress of an action comes to a standstill
Digress	Going away from main point
Diplomacy	Art of negotiations at international level
Drought	Dry and unproductive area due to failure of rain
Democracy	Government by the people, for the people
Dubious	False statement shown as true statement
Edible	Food fit for human consumption
Egoist	Self-centred man
Eligible	Qualified for selection
Emigrant	Person who has come to settle in another country
Encyclopaedia	Huge authoritative book which gives all required information
Epicure	Person fond of luxury who can appreciate good food and drink

Epilogue	Concluding part of a literary work
Epidemic	Diseases occurring everywhere and more than our expectations
Epitaph	Words inscribed on a tomb about a buried man
Extempore	Speaking without preparation
Ecology	Environment that influences the living of man
Egoist	Person always thinks of himself as supreme
Executive	One who carries out the law or policy made
Elucidate	Explaining mysterious or difficult items
Emphasis	Lay special stress on a thing
Eradicate	Taking out the root of diseases in man Taking out the root of an evil in society
Equilibrium	State of perfect balance
Exile	Punishing a person by sending out of his country or state
Fanatic	Excessive and mistaken enthusiasm on religion
Fauna	Animals existing in a geographical area
Fatalist	Person believing about fate
Feminist	Champions the claims of women
Fission	Splitting of the nucleus of an atom
Flora	Plants existing in a geographical area
Fastidious	Person who is not pleased easily or fussy
Galaxy	Stars encircling the heavens
Genealogy	Description of a person's descent from his ancestors
Geology	Natural science dealing with earth's strata and crust
Gravitation	Natural attractive force which pulls all material towards the centre of the earth
Gymnasium	Equipped place for the practice of physical exercises
Glutton	One who eats too much
Hallucination	Seeing, hearing or tasting which does not exist
Hedonist	Person living only for pleasure
Hereditary	Characteristics descending from parents to offspring
Honorary	Serving without any expectation of money or material
Horticulture	Art of garden cultivation
Hypothesis	Supposition made as a basis for reasoning in research
Homicide	Murder of a person for a gain
Humanitarian	Sympathetic towards other fellowmen
Idealism	Practise and following of the ideals

Ideology	Ideas based on economic and political system
Illiterate	One who is not able to read and write
Immemorial	That which is too old to be remembered
Immigrant	One who comes as a permanent resident
Imminent	That which is about to happen
Immunity	Body resistance not to develop infection
Inaudible	That cannot be heard
Inaugural	That which is connected with opening ceremony
Inauspicious	Not of good omen
Inevitable	That which cannot be avoided
Infectious	The disease which spreads to others easily through some means
Intolerable	That cannot be tolerated
Introspection	Visualisation of one's own mental make up
Intuition	Getting apprehended without reasoning
Invalid	Made null and void
Invincible	That which cannot be conquered
Isthmus	Narrow neck which connects two big items
Immovable	Item which cannot be moved
Insolvent	One who is unable to pay one's debts
Impracticable	That which cannot be put into practice
Illicit	A business that is prohibited by government or law
Irrelevant	A remark that cannot apply to present discussion
Inflammable	Liable to catch fire easily
Invisible	That which is not visible to naked eye
Irritable	One who gets angry easily.
Incorrigible	Person who cannot be corrected
Idiosyncrasy	The temperament is peculiar in a person
Journalism	The science that deals with editing and writing news or article
Judicious	If it is sound in judgement
Jurisdiction	Boundary for the authority for an individual
Kennel	Small dog house where watchdogs are placed in front of the house
Laissez faire	Government do not interfere in trade, commerce or industry
Lethal	That which is made to cause death
Lunar	Related to the moon
Migratory	Seasonal migration of birds from one country to another
Mediate	Negotiation to settle the differences
Menu	Details of food available in a restaurant
Misogamist	Person who hates marriage

Monogamy	Practising one or single marriage in lifetime
Monopoly	Exclusive possession of trade by one person
Mortuary	Place where dead bodies are kept for autopsy or for waiting for near relative to come and take
Museum	Place where art, sculpture, objects and antiquities are exhibited
Nepotism	Favour shown by a person in power to his relatives
Neurotic	Person who suffers from nervous disorder
Neutral	One who remains impartial
Nucleus	That which can receive addition Central portion of an atom
Obituary	Notice given of a person's death
Observatory	Building from where stars and planets are watched through telescope
Omnipotent	That which has infinite or unimaginable power
Omnipresent	Having the power to be present everywhere, referred to God
Omniscient	Having infinite knowledge
Optimist	Person who looks towards the bright aspect of happening
Orbit	Circular and curved path of planet where they rotate through it
Oligarchy	Government by small group of powerful people
Orthodox	Person who holds the established opinions Obsolete. That which is no longer in use
Opportunist	Shaping his fortune according to circumstances, taking advantages of the moment
Panacea	Remedy that cures all illness
Panorama	Unbroken view of surrounding region
Paradox	Statement contradictory to accepted opinion
Passport	Legal permission document to travel outside the country
Patent	Sole right and ownership to produce and sell some invention
Perquisite	Additional profit over and above one's own salary
Pessimist	Person who looks at the dark side of events
Polygamy	Marrying many wives seen in certain religion and in tribal community
Portable	That which can be easily transported
Posthumous	That which occurs after the death of an individual

Pseudonym	Name used as fictitious one by an author
Plutocracy	Government by the rich
Polyandry	Woman marrying more than one husband
Plagiarist	Ideas and words are borrowed by a writer
Philanthropist	Person who is the lover of mankind
Physiology	Science which deals with functions of human body
Pathology	Science which deals with gross and microscopic changes that occurs in disease or illness
Pharmacology	Science which deals with drugs used in the treatment of illness
Philistine	Uncultured person whose interests are purely material and common place
Post mortem	Inspection and examination of body for the cause of death, done after the death of a person
Paediatrician	Specialist who treats the illness of children
Partiality	Tendency to give unfair judgement through sympathy with one side
Precedent	Earlier incident which can serve as an example
Quintessence	Purest and most essential aspect of a considered thing
Radar	Instrument used to find out the range of aircraft or warships
Radioactive	Capable of producing spontaneous powerful rays
Redtapism	Unnecessary delay due to official formalities
Regime	Existing system to run the government
Reinforce	Strengthen by additional manpower and material
Reinstate	Restoring the lost job or position
Sabotage	Wanton destruction of animal, plant or substance
Sarcasm	Hurting with ironically used words
Scapegoat	Person who is made to bear the blame due to others
Sceptic	Person who doubts the truth of religion and religious doctrines
Scion	Young member of royal family
Sculpture	Carving figures in wood, marble, stone or metal
Silhouette	Black shadow like picture on white background
Simultaneous	Events happening at the same time in different places

Söjourn	Short stay of a person in a place before reaching distant place
Soliloquy	Loud thinking and loud speaking alone
Solo	Music or musical instrument played by a single person
Spendthrift	Person who spends money extravagantly
Spinster	An unmarried woman
Stable	Place where horses are kept
Stampede	Sudden rush of people or animals due to some frightening event
Superfluous	More than that is necessary
Samaritan	Person who helps a helpless in difficulties
Somnambulism	One who walks in sleep
Spokesperson	Representative meant to speak for his party or for his group
Sacrilege	Destroying the property of sacred place
Superstition	Irrational and ignorant belief of a person or of a society
Tableau	Scene represented by silent and motionless people
Teetotaller	One who never uses liquor
Transmigration	Soul passing to another body after death of a person according to a belief
Truant	Child who stays away from school without leave
Temporary	That which lasts for a short time
Transparent	Capable of being seen through
Ultimatum	Final warning given to a party by the government or by terrorists
Unanimous	Being all of one opinion
Upstart	Sudden rising of a person from low rank to high rank and to importance
Utopian	Perfect and ideal but imaginary and impossible
Voluntary	Acting at one's own will and wish
Vacillate	To waver in opinion or resolution
Verbose	Style full of words wanted or unwanted
Vindicate	Establish the justice of a cause
Veteran	One who has long experience of any occupation
Vegetarian	One who eats only vegetarian food
Windfall	Expected occurrence of good fortune
Witticism	Amusing but clever saying
Zenith	Highest point in the sky
Zoo	Place where animals are kept for show

7.4. WORDS OFTEN CONFUSED

Students often make mistakes with certain words which are same by pronunciations but differ in their spellings. Context gets defective if care is not taken.

They should make an effort to use them repeatedly in their usage if they want to master over these terminologies.

Their meanings are given in the following table:

Spelling	*Substance*	*Spelling*	*Substance*
Affect	to act upon	Effect	to bring about
Adverse	hostile	Averse	dislike
Accelerate	increase speed	Expedite	hasten the progress
Application	to apply	Implication	mean, not explicate
Ancient	very old	Antique	old fashioned
Apprehend	to grasp	Comprehend	fully understand
Assent	sanction	Ascent	climb up
Amiable	lovable	Amicable	friendly
Adapt	made suitable	Adopt	taking into relation
Apposite	relevant	Opposite	contrary
Allusion	reference	Illusion	false notion
Abstract	brief summary	Extract	passage taken
Avert	ward off	Invert	to turn upside down
Attenuate	to make thin	Extenuate	to diminish
Accept	to receive	Except	to exclude
Aught	any thing	Ought	should
Advise	verb (to advise)	Advice	noun (the advice)
Affection	love	Affectation	pretending
Artist	singer, dramatist	Artisan	useful crafts doing
Accede	agree	Exceed	be greater than
Beside	by the side of	Besides	in addition to
Beneficial	useful	Beneficent	kind
Bridal	wedding	Bridle	control
Canvas	cloth for tent	Canvass	request vote
Council	advisers	Counsel	advice
Corporal	physical	Corporate	body politic
Continual	frequent	Continuous	unceasing

Contd.

Contd.

Childlike	like a child	Childish	immature
Congenial	agreeable	Congenital	since birth
Capture	seize	Captivate	fascinate
Collision	violent contact	Collusion	secret under-standing
Compliment	express regard	Complement	full number
Confident	sure	Confidential	secret
Confirm	ratify	Conform	comply with
Contagious	spread by contact	Contiguous	adjoining
Dependent	adjective (depend)	Dependant	noun (person)
Destiny	fate	Destination	goal
Dual	double	Duel	a combat
Disease	illness	Decease	death
Eligible	qualified	Illegible	unreadable
Elusive	evading	Illusive	deceptive
Emigrate	leave country	Immigrate	to come to country
Eminent	illustrious	Imminent	about to happen
Estimate	calculated	Estimation	opinion
Facilitate	make easy	Felicitate	congratulate
Flagrant	glaring	Fragrant	sweet smelling
Imaginary	not real	Imaginative	gifted to imagine
Industrial	industry related	Industrious	hard work
Ingenuous	frank	Ingenious	clever
Judicial	legal	Judicious	prudent
Junction	meeting place	Juncture	grave situation
Momentary	for a moment	Momentous	important
Masterful	imperious	Masterly	skilful
Metal	iron like	Mettle	courage
Official	of an office	Officious	unwanted service
Popular	liked	Populous	thickly populated
Principal	chief	Principle	general law
Stationary	motionless	Stationery	writing material
Verbal	word related	Verbose	wordy
Wave	brandish	Waive	relinquish

Chapter 8

Conversation

Conversation is "**informal spoken communication**". The origin is from French related to converse, as a verb meaning "to talk".

English is called universal language. Using this language, speaking and conversing with people around the world is possible. When you are talking with anybody around you, say with a friend, a teacher, an examiner, a patient or with a doctor on duty, you should keep up fluency. Fluency comes with confidence. This is possible by various means. One such means could be to think in English and then to speak in English. By doing so your conversation will not have breaks and will not mar the fluency. Think in mother tongue to speak in English is also advocated.

When you are talking in English, try to remember pronunciations and grammar. These will enhance your standard of conversation.

If English was mother tongue, the child would have learnt colloquial way of talking. But speaking English in India needs good learning. This is made possible by giving opportunity to children to speak in English with known people. This will help to converse with another individual or with a group of people.

But, all said and done, conversation sometimes becomes colloquial in its occurrence. This will not deter your talk or vocabulary. Make the speaking meaningful and have substance in the conversation.

Proficiency in spoken English will enhance your status in the society.

Following are the key points in acquiring skill in a good conversation:

- Speak logically.
- Have clear idea for expression.
- Talk in a familiar manner.
- Avoid unnecessary interruption.
- Use interjections for surprises that gives weightage.
- Let it be realistic.
- Let it be interesting and never be boring.
- Let it be natural and never be artificial.

8.1. CONVERSATION WITH A FRIEND

Conversation between Rita and Shobha, Final B.Sc. Nursing students

Rita	How did you write the Final Examination?
Shobha	I have written extremely well Rita. I am sure of getting above 85% in the examination. By the way, how you have done?
Rita	I have written average Shobha. I may get through. Well, what do you do if you get high first class in the Final Examination?
Shobha	I want to join M.Sc. Nursing. What about you?
Rita	I will not study further. My father is a General Practitioner. I will help him in his clinic.
Shobha	Rekha was telling that she has not done well in the examination and that she may fail. Is it so doubtful?
Rita	Yes. She hasn't done well. She absented from class for over four months owing to her marriage and hence could not study well.
Shobha	Our new tutor wanted to go abroad for her nursing career there. Any progress in her venture?
Rita	She has succeeded in her venture. Nowadays there is great demand for

	nursing career abroad like U S A, U K, Canada, Saudi Arabia and other Gulf Countries. They welcome Indian Nurses for job, offering high perks.
Shobha	By the way, how to go about this type of employment abroad?
Rita	First, you should apply to concerned hospital. You should get selected through interview. You need passport and visa to go abroad.
Shobha	If we have some one, we could have tried.
Rita	Alright let the results be announsed. We shall see to the other things afterwards.

8.2. CONVERSATION WITH A TEACHER

(Conversation between Tutor and Student Nurse on the day of the latter's joining)

Tutor	Which is your native place?
Student nurse	I am from Hassan, which is a district in Karnataka.
Tutor	What is your father?
Student nurse	He is a school teacher at Hassan and we have a house at Hassan.
Tutor	Tell me about the members of your family at Hassan.
Student nurse	My father, mother, elder brother, sister-in-law and their child live in that house.
Tutor	You have joined B.Sc. nursing course. Where will you stay?
Student nurse	I will stay in the hostel provided by you.
Tutor	You must follow regulations of the hostel and should be in the hostel by 7.00 PM every day.
Student nurse	Madam, what should be done when I have ward duty at night?
Tutor	You are permitted to stay in the ward since you are posted for the duty.
Student nurse	It is nice madam.

Tutor	When you go out of the hostel on holidays, you should inform warden and leave the message of your expected time of returns as well as the place of visit.
Student nurse	Yes madam. I will inform warden.
Tutor	OK you can go now. I wish you all the best.
Student nurse	Thank you madam.

8.3. CONVERSATION WITH EXAMINER

(Conversation between the Examiner and the Student Nurse)

Examiner	Good morning, come in, be seated.
Student nurse	Thank you madam.
Examiner	What is your roll number in the examination?
Student nurse	KA 25 M 3076
Examiner	What are the indications of Per Vaginal Examination?
Student nurse	It is done for the purpose of diagnosis, for smear taking and as pre operative examination.
Examiner	Good. Name the speculum used in PV examination.
Student nurse	Ferguson's Speculum.
Examiner	Name the forceps used in PV examination.
Student nurse	It is Vulsellum Forceps.
Examiner	Very good. Name a few paired organs in our body.
Student nurse	Eyes, Kidneys.
Examiner	OK. Any other paired organs?
Student nurse	(Just thinking, not answering).
Tutor	All right, we respire through which organs? And what operation is done for family planning in women?
Student nurse	Yes, madam, I got the clue. They are Lungs and Fallopian tubes.

Tutor	That is good. Let me ask you a last question. Tell me what special nursing care do you give in severe malaria of a child?
Student nurse	The special nursing care in severe malaria of a child include the following: Correction of hypoglycaemia; Restoring circulating volume; and Treatment of anaemia.
Tutor	Well, to prevent aspiration pneumonia, what will you do?
Student nurse	Madam, nasogastric tube is to be inserted.
Tutor	Excellent. You have answered well. Do well in other practical. You can go.
Student nurse	Thank you madam.

8.4. CONVERSATION WITH PATIENT

8.4.1. Conversation with a Patient in Medical Ward

(Conversation between the nurse and a patient)

Patient	Sister, I am not well.
Nurse	What health problem do you have?
Patient	I find it hard to spend time during night due to sleeplessness, I feel weak and I have pain in my left leg.
Nurse	OK, Tell me your name, age, place of residence and complaints. I shall fill the case sheet.
Patient	Yes sister.
Nurse	What is your age?
Patient	59 years.
Nurse	Which is your native place?
Patient	I am from Shiggaon.
Nurse	How is your appetite?
Patient	I always feel hungry.
Nurse	Your weight is 82 kgs. and it is overweight. You need other investigations

	in our laboratory. Of course, your B.P. is normal.
Patient	Why I get pain in my leg?
Nurse	You may be having arthritis. Let us see what doctors say.
Patient	OK sister.
Nurse	Your body weight is more. You must be put on a therapeutic diet to reduce your overweight.
Patient	Sister, I was examined by the doctor. He has prescribed tablets to be taken 3 times a day.
Nurse	Good. Follow the doctor's advice.
Patient	Sister, doctor has advised me to cut down the calorie. How can I do?
Nurse	Take this chart which gives you the Therapeutic diet for reducing weight. Since you are a non-vegetarian, you are given the chart which shows Low Calorie weight reducing diet for Non-vegetarian. Look, doctor has instructed me to tell you the foods you should avoid and the foods which are allowed liberally. Foods to avoid are—whole milk, cream, butter, oils, ghee, fried foods and honey. Sugar, sweets of all kinds, ovaltine, horlicks, cocoa and cheese. Banana, mangoes, grapes, jam, arvi and potatoes. All aerated water except soda. Alcohols. Dried fruit and nuts. Foods allowed liberally are—all vegetables, lime juice, clear soups and pepper water. Skimmed milk and its preparations. All fruits.
Patient	Thank you sister for these details. What else I should follow?
Nurse	Have 2 kilometres walk every day to keep you fit.
Patient	Thank you sister.
Nurse	OK. Take care of your health and come after one week for follow-up.

8.4.2. Conversation with patient in Dental Ward

(Conversation between the nurse and a patient)

Nurse	Your teeth are caries teeth and with cavities. Hence you are suffering from pain.
Patient	Should I have to get this extracted?
Nurse	Let us see what Dentists advice. Open your mouth.
Patient	Yes sister (Opens his mouth).
Nurse	It needs filling. Do you get it filled with gold or by cement?
Patient	Cement is OK sister.
Nurse	Your gum is swollen. Even that needs check-up by the Dentist.
Patient	OK sister.
Nurse	Which tooth paste you use?
Patient	I do not use tooth paste and I use tooth powder. How much is charged for tooth extraction?
Nurse	Rs. 25/- per tooth is charged.
Patient	Will it be painful?
Nurse	No. Doctor will give injection to anaesthetise the area during tooth extraction.
Patient	Sister, Dentist has extracted my painful tooth. Now it is bleeding.
Nurse	Open your mouth. I keep a swab. Hold it for some time. Bleeding will stop.
Patient	Can I go home now?
Nurse	No. Stay for another 30 minutes since I want to observe you as per doctor's instruction. Later you can go.
Patient	What advise should I follow for my dental care?
Nurse	Brush your teeth before going to bed. Do not smoke Do not take too hot or too cold water or food. Rinse your mouth after eating sweet.

Patient	Thank you sister for your valuable advice.
Nurse	OK, Take this receipt for Rs. 25/- towards doctor's fee for your tooth extraction.
Patient	Thank you.

8.5. CONVERSATION WITH DOCTOR ON DUTY

(Conversation between the nurse and the doctor on duty)

Doctor	Sister, get the case to emergency resuscitation room. It is mild heart attack case.
Nurse	I have put him on the resuscitation table. I gave Pethidine injection. Patient is now feeling comfortable doctor.
Doctor	Check his pulse, B.P. and respiratory rate.
Nurse	I have checked pulse. It is 86 per minute regular and normal tone. B.P. is 110/70 mm of Hg (millimetre of mercury) and his respiratory rate is 21 per minute but regular doctor.
Doctor	Sister; send words to ECG (Electro Cardio Graphy) technician for taking an ECG. It is very urgent.
Nurse	Yes doctor.
Doctor	E.C.G. shows mild heart attack. Patient must be totally in bed rest till he recovers. Shift him to ICCU (Intensive Coronary Care Unit).
Nurse	Doctor, patient's relatives are disturbed. What advice should I give to them?
Doctor	Tell them that patient has mild heart attack which is called Myocardial Infarction. Blood circulation to the heart is impaired. Since patient has come in time he will have 100%

	recovery. But tell them they cannot see the patient since it disturbs his complete rest.
Nurse	OK doctor. I will convey to his relatives.
Doctor	I have written doctor's advice in case sheet. Let this be followed scrupulously.
Nurse	Yes doctor. Doctor, can the patient have something to drink if he asks?
Doctor	No. Nothing is allowed till he is settled in ICCU. Shift him immediately and report to me.
Nurse	Yes doctor. It is done.
Doctor	You have come back to casualty from ICCU. How is that patient?
Nurse	He is comfortable and is sleeping due to the effect of drug. Ward sister will be informing his progress over intercom sir.
Doctor	OK thank you sister.

Chapter 9 Nursing Terminology

Abdomen It is the cavity between diaphragm and the pelvis. It is colloquially called *belly.*

Abortion Foetus is expelled before it is viable. Types are complete abortion, incomplete abortion, threatened abortion, induced abortion, missed abortion, septic abortion, therapeutic abortion, inevitable abortion, criminal abortion and tubal abortion.

Abscess It is a collection of pus in a cavity.

Abstinence Denial of indulgence in food, alcohol, drink and sex.

Acetone Blood and urine contain traces of acetone. Chemically it is a colourless inflammable liquid with characteristic odour. Increased in starvation and diabetes.

Acid burn Corrosive acid burns are severe. Comes under special varieties of burns.

Acid Fast Bacteria causing tuberculosis and leprosy are acid fast bacilli, because they are not decolourised by mineral acids after staining.

Acromegaly Gigantism, over activity of anterior lobe of pituitary gland.

Adenoid Hypertrophy of pharyngeal tonsil present in children. Any structure which resembles a gland.

Adolescence Period of life when physical growth and secondary sexual characteristics appear.

Air Embolism	Sudden blocking of an artery or a vein by air, a risk in I.V. infusion or trauma to jugular vein.
Albinism	A clinical condition where skin pigment is lost, sometimes changes in hair or in eyes are seen.
Alternative medicine	Holistic approach of medical treatment which consists of homoeopathy, aromatherapy, hypnosis, acupuncture etc.
Allergy	Hypersensitive state produced by the exposure to an allergen.
Amine	Any organic compound containing nitrogen, according to number of hydrogen atoms replaced. They are termed primary, secondary and tertiary amines. E.g., allylamine, phenylamine, propylamine.
Amnesia	Loss of memory.
Amputation	Surgical removal of an organ or a limb.
Anaemia	Quality or quantity of RBC is deficient. Types are microcytic anaemia, hypochromic anaemia, macrocytic anaemia, aplastic anaemia, haemolytic anaemia, pernicious anaemia, sickle cell anaemia.
Anastomosis	Surgical formation or pathological formation of a passage.
Aneurysm	Local distension and dilation of an artery. Types are dissecting saccular and fusiform aneurysms.
Apnoea	Cessation of respiration, Types are cardiac apnoea, sleep apnoea and prematurity apnoea.
Apoplexy	Stroke due to rupture of cerebral artery.
Appendicitis	Infection and inflammation of appendix, usually an acute condition, may be chronic in nature.
Aspermia	Absence of sperm in the semen.

Astigmatism Ray of light is not sharply focused on the retina, diffused image is focussed, seen either vertical or horizontal at a point of time.

Asthma Dyspnoea with wheezing and difficulty in expiration; difficulty in breathing as in allergy.

Atherosclerosis Lesion of medium and large sized arteries with plaques of lipoid material and cholesterol in intima.

Atrophy Malnourishment, degeneration or disuse leads to wasting of a tissue.

Autoimmune disease Clinical condition where ones own body develops antibody against its tissue culminating in self destruction.

Autopsy Post-mortem examination of dead to establish the cause of death, medico legal procedure.

Bag technique Bag made of canvas, leather or light metal is used in home visiting. Specifications are made for bag and its content for use by the public health nurse who visits families for primary health care.

Bed making A nursing skill to suit the bed to the sick, clean smooth linens, covers of the right warmth for the season, protective rubber pads, making one half of the bed while the patient lies on the other, rolling the patient gently to the made up side and finishing up the other.

Bimanual Examination done by using both hands, gynaecological examination, examination by one hand on abdomen and the other in the vagina for internal genital organs.

Bio nursing Biology knowledge is used in nursing practice.

Biopsy Surgical removal of tissue for diagnosis.

Bland diet	Diet which do not contain spices or hard foodstuffs, a therapeutic diet.
Blue baby	Cyanosis of the newborn due to congenital malformation of the heart.
Broxton Hicks Contraction	A test for detection of meningeal irritation, flexion of one thigh causes the flexion of other thigh, flexion of neck causes bilateral flexion of hips and knees.
Buerger's disease	Other name for thrombo angiitis obliterans.
Burkitt's tumour	African lymphoma a lymphosarcoma
Crohn's disease	A chronic condition of the terminal portion of the ileum in which granulation and oedema may give rise to obstruction.
Cachexia	Severe debility, commonly late stage of illness. severe malnutrition. severe muscular wasting.
Caisson disease	It is decompression sickness, found in people working in low altitude with high atmospheric pressure, in lower altitude with high atmospheric pressure gases are in liquid form; if air pressure is rapidly reduced it produces symptoms due to bubbling out of dissolved nitrogen, it is also called *diver's disease.*
Carbuncle	Acute staphylococcal infection of subcutaneous tissues multiple boils which tend to undermine the skin.
Cell	Smallest unit of living organism which go to form tissue.
Cervicitis	Infection and inflammation of cervix.
Cheyne Stokes respiration	Colloquially it is called tidal respiration, it is irregular rhythmic breathing with temporary apnoea, causes are narcotic poisoning, arteriosclerosis, uraemia and cerebral tumours.

Cholera	Acute intestinal infection caused by *Vibrio cholerae* bacteria, it is notifiable disease, it is quarantinable disease.
Chorea	Spasmodic involuntary rapid movements of face, hip and shoulder which is due to pathology of basal ganglion, two clinical entities of chorea are seen in practice. One is Huntington's chorea in middle age and is hereditary and the other is Sydenham's chorea in children and is called St.Vitus dance.
Chromosome	Main component of cell which contain genetic information.
Coarctation	Stricture or constriction of vessels as seen in coarctation of aorta.
Colitis	Infection and inflammation of colon due to various reasons, inflammatory changes in large bowel, emotional and bacterial causes are known.
Collagen disease	They are types of rheumatic diseases; collagen is applied to the term connective tissue of the body such as bursitis, fibrositis, tenosynovitis and lumbago.
Convulsion	It is the state of involuntary contraction of voluntary muscles due to organic causes or sometimes by unknown causes, common clinical types are major convulsion and minor convulsion. Unconsciousness accompanied by muscular twitching.
Coronary thrombosis	Clot formation and blocking of coronary artery which cause angina pectoris and M.I.
Cri du chat syndrome	It is a chromosomal disorder characterised by microcephaly, mental retardation, dwarfism and laryngeal defect with cat's cry.
Cytoplasm	Fluid present in the cell.
Darling's disease	Histoplasmosis is known as Darling's disease.

Deerfly fever Other name for tularaemia.

Dehydration State of loss of fluid from the body, common causes are vomiting, diarrhoea and Sweating. Shock and acidosis are its sequelae.

Dementia Irreversible changes in mental acumen which give rise to loss of memory, loss of judgement, loss of emotional control. Varieties are senile dementia, presenile dementia, atherosclerotic dementia, Alzheimer's disease, Creutzfeldt Jakob disease and Loss of memory due to brain pathological changes or senescence.

Dermatitis Infection and inflammation of skin tissue; depending upon the cause of dermatitis we have contact dermatitis, X-ray dermatitis, varicose dermatitis, traumatic dermatitis, allergic dermatitis, occupational dermatitis and exfoliative dermatitis.

Desert fever Other name for coccidioidomycosis.

Diabetes Disturbance of glucose metabolism due to malfunction of beta cells of pancreas. Type I and Type II are common clinical types.

Diarrhoea Frequent evacuation of loose stool which bring about body changes due to dehydration, loose water stool which is passed frequently which can cause body dehydration and salt loss.

Dirt eating It is called pica a bad habit among children who eat dirt. Historically the word has come from Latin which refers to a bird that eats everything unfit for food—magpie; since mouth is main organ of tactile sensing child gets to dirt eating.

Disinfection To take away infection by means of available measures like physical disinfectants, chemical disinfectants and common types of disinfection are

	prophylactic disinfection, concurrent disinfection and terminal disinfection.
Dislocation	Displacement of a bone on to other bone which is also called subluxation or luxation.
Disorientation	Mental confusion for place, time and person; person who cannot identify or has confusion with regard to time and place where he stands.
Diuretics	They are medications which increase the amount of urine secretion from the kidneys.
DOTS	It is a strategy to ensure cure by providing most effective drug and confirming that the drug is taken. It strands for directly observed treatment short course.
Douche	To flush out a cavity, permitted fluids are used as flushing agent, vaginal irrigations are done for preoperative cleansing with providone iodine solution for smoothening inflamed vaginal mucosa and for applying medications to the vaginal mucosa.
Drip	IV infusion of fluid in case of dehydration or sickness.
Dysmenorrhoea	Clinical condition depicting painful menses, two common types are primary and secondary.
Eale's disease	Thrombophlebitis of retinal vein causing retinal haemorrhage and vitreous haemorrhage an auto immune disease.
Ecchymosis	A skin discolouration caused by effusion of blood below the skin due to a bruise.
Eczema	Superficial inflammation of epidermis which is staged by redness, papule, vesicle, crusting and scaling, allergic dermatitis is called atopic dermatitis, chronic skin lesion due to allergic origin.

Elephantiasis	Swelling in scrotum, leg, penis, breast, hand etc., due to lymphatic stasis secondary to filarial infection; hypertrophy of skin and subcutaneous tissue occurs.
Eligible couple	They are women in the age group of 15 to 45 years of age from whom following couples are excluded – primary sterility, secondary sterility and early menopause.
Embolism	A loose blood clot which is in the circulation, which when blocks a vessel may cause partial or complete block and an emergency.
Emphysema	Presence of air in a cavity or in a tissue which is abnormal or pathological; surgical emphysema and pulmonary emphysema are known.
Encephalitis	Infection and inflammation of the brain, that can be septic, tubercular or parasitic in nature.
Endocarditis	Inflammation of the endocardium due to infection by bacteria, fungus or rickettsia infection and inflammation of inner lining membrane of the heart.
Enzyme	Organic substance helping digestion and metabolism.
Epilepsy	A neurological disorder which is primarily a disease of brain which can cause grand mal or petit mal (major fits and minor fits).
Epulis	It is a tumour of lower jaw which is fibrous, sarcomatous in nature.
Erb's palsy	When birth injury or assisted delivery causes injury it causes pressure on cervical nerve or brachial plexus that produces paralysis of the arm in the new born.
Erythema	Abnormal condition of skin with fearful redness of the skin due to local congestion, common causes being sunburn and inflammation.

Essential new born care	Under RCH this component is intended to reduce perinatal and neonatal mortality in the community; this includes: resuscitation of newborn with birth asphyxia, prevention of hypothermia, prevention of infection, exclusive breastfeeding, referral of sick newborn and care of low birth weight babies.
Essential obstetrical care	This refers to basic maternity service to all pregnant women in the country to ensure registration of pregnancy at 16th week, 3 antenatal check ups by ANM, safe delivery either at home or at health centre and 3 post natal check- ups.
Etiology	Cause of an illness.
Exanthema	Skin rashes occurring in case of infectious diseases
Fallot's tetralogy	It is a congenital heart disease with the defects of Pulmonary stenosis, VSD, Overriding of the aorta and hypertrophy of the right ventricle.
Fat embolism	This is a common complication of severe trauma with multiple fractures, Hip fracture and femur fracture should be followed for minimum 3 days to exclude fat embolism. Early signs of fat embolism are raised temperature, increased pulse rate, precordial chest pain, dyspnoea, cough, agitation and disorientation.
Fever	The body temperature is elevated than normal, sometimes seen in conjunction with identified fevers like dengue fever, typhoid fever.
Filaria	One of the nematodes that cause elephantiasis, also called filariasis.
Fistula	That which connects two cavities of two organs, abnormal passage formed between surfaces. Such as recto vaginal fistula, anal fistula etc.

Furuncle Other name for boil which is manifested due to staphylococcal infection.

GAD Generalised Anxiety Disorder is characterised by persistent anxiety expressed by tachycardia, choking, dry mouth dyspepsia, urinary frequency and body pain.

Gene It is a hereditary unit.

Geriatric nursing Nursing care of the elderly in hospital, health centre, old age home. Elderly people in their home call for nursing care from nursing profession, along with clinical rehabilitation, home visiting is demanded by the community.

Glioma Tumour of neuroglial cells in brain and spinal cord.

Glomerulo-nephritis Disease affecting the glomerules which perform the main kidney function probably of immune origin leading to inflammation of glomeruli and kidney causing acute and or chronic clinical condition.

Gonorrhoea It is sexually transmitted disease caused by N. gonorrhoeae infecting genital tract causing discharge and pain during urination.

Gout A general disease where body cannot handle protein foods containing purine bodies. Excess uric acid in blood causing swelling and inflammation of toes and fingers.

Haasim This is the nickname given to some of the clinical conditions among children such as bleeding disorders, stoppage of breathing, lung collapse, severe sepsis, syphilis manifestations, severe jaundice, and meningeal irritations.

Haematoma Due to injury or a slow bleeding under the skin occur although no actual wound has been caused, soft swelling formed thus is haematoma.

Haemophilia	It is a hereditary hypo prothrombinaemia which causes bleeding tendencies among males who inherit the disease from their mothers. It is called Royal disease.
Haemoptysis	Bright red and frothy blood is coughed out from lung and bronchi which is due to lung pathology like cancer, gastric ulcers.
Haemorrhoids	Varicosity of rectal veins, colloquially called piles at or above the anus.
Hallucination	Seeing, hearing or experiencing a thing which is not there in the true sense.
Hansen's disease	A chronic bacterial disease caused by M. leprae.
Heart block	There is an interruption in AV node which leads to independent beating of auricles and ventricles.
Heat exhaustion	When a person collapses due to overexposure to heat. Pale, clammy skin, rapid and weak pulse, weakness, head- ache and nausea are common.
Heat stroke	It is a severe form of reaction to exposure of man to hot climate. Flushed hot skin, rapid and strong pulse are seen.
Helminthiasis	Intestinal infection with helminths like cystode, trematodes and nematodes which are due to poor personal and environmental hygiene.
Hemiplegia	One side of the body is paralysed due to cerebral haemorrhage.
Hepatitis	Infection and inflammation of liver by different types of viruses and by toxic agents including alcohol.
Hernia	In a weak body structure organs are pushed into areas where they do not belong such as inguinal hernia, umbilical hernia etc.
Herpes	Skin eruptions by herpes viral infection commonly occurring in mucocutaneous junction of lip and vagina.

Hiccough Sharp inspiratory cough which follows the closure of glottis and spasmodic contraction of diaphragm.

Home nursing Public health nursing leads to the care of the sick at home by the special nurse who attends to him or her in their surroundings; in case of communicable diseases, Parkinson's disease, stroke, cancer and certain chronic disorders need home nursing care.

Huntington chorea It is an inherited disorder of nervous system which give rise to dementia.

Hydrocele In tunica vaginalis when fluid accumulates, it is called hydrocele.

Hydramnios Clinically it is called polyhydramnios. Anatomically defined when liquor amnii exceeds 2000 ml: clinically defined when it causes discomfort: sonographically defined when AFI (Amniotic Fluid Index) is more than 20 cm.

Hypertension High blood pressure which is usually pathological. In an individual if BP is persistently high at supine arterial systolic greater than 140 mmHg and diastolic lies greater than 90 mmHg (when resting and taken on three consecutive days in early morning) hypertension is diagnosed.

Hyperthyroidism Hyperactivity of thyroid gland giving rise to clinical conditions which include thyrotoxicosis.

Hypothermia Is due to fall in body temperature since ambient temperature to which they are born is always by several degrees cooler than temperature in the womb.

Hysteria Lack of control over acts and emotions called psychoneurosis.

Iatrogenic Infections, new reactions, side effects and psychological distress because of complications, rare medicaments,

	drugs and activities of health professionals are called iatrogenic effects.
Impairment	Usually referred to vision and hearing, if structural and functional changes in an organ. Psychological abnormality, loss of structure or function or both.
Impotence	It usually refers to absence or failure of sexual function in male.
Infantile paralysis	This is the colloquial name for poliomyelitis a viral infection in the community which produce paralysis among infants.
Infarction	It refers to the formation of an infarct. It is called heart attack.
Inflammation	Reaction of cell or tissue to injury or infection, marked by redness, pain, swelling and heat.
ICU	Intensive care unit, an established unit for the treatment of critically ill.
Ishihara chart	Chart devised by a Japanese Ophthalmologist contains patterns of dots of primary colours on similar background which a normal man can see whereas a colour blind cannot see them.
IVF	In Vitro Fertilisation colloquially called 'test tube baby'.
Jaundice	Bile pigment in the blood and tissues giving them a yellow appearance, liver disorders, icterus.
Juvenile delinquency	Disorder and disruption caused by young in a society.
Kala azar	Tropical leishmania infection transmitted by sand fly.
Keratomalacia	Softening of the cornea in vitamin A deficiency, cause of preventable blindness.
KFD	Kyasanur Forest Disease. Prevailing only in Karnataka state, called monkey fever transmitted by hard tick.

Kidney stone	Urate, oxalate or phosphates of calcium stone present in renal parenchyma; gout and hyper function of parathyroid usually stimulate kidney stone formation.
Koch's bacilli	This bacteria causes tuberculosis.
Koplik' spot	Its presence is pathognomonic of measles, spots on internal buccal mucosa.
Kussmaul's Breathing	Acidosis, deep and gasping respiration in acidosis
Kwashiorkor	Local name of Africa meaning 'golden boy'. Protein deficiency disorder among underprivileged children.
Kyphosis	Humpback appearance of a man because of bend in spinal curvature.
Labour	Process of childbirth which is described in 3 stages.
Landsteiner's Classification	A system of blood grouping into O, A, B and AB.
Last offices	Procedures that are followed when death of patient takes place.
Leg cramps	In pregnant women, because of impaired circulation muscle spasms occur which can be relieved by nursing procedure and exercise.
Leptospirosis	Jaundice because of leptospiral infection in man.
Lipid	Organic compound containing fats and oil.
Lordosis	Exaggerated forward curve of lumbar area.
Low birth weight	When birth weight of newborn is below 2500 grams prevalence is 30% in developing countries.
Lupus erythematosus	Inflammatory changes in skin and internal organs in autoimmune disorders.
MI	Abbreviation for Myocardial infarction (heart attack).
Macmillan nurses	Trained nurses in pain relief and palliative care of cancer patients.

Malaria	Protozoal infection caused by Plasmodium malarial parasite which is transmitted by anopheles mosquito.
Malta fever	Native name for brucellosis.
Malthusian theory	Postulates that over population is controlled by natural calamities like volcano, earthquake, floods, epidemics etc.
Marasmus	Manifestation of PEM found infants and children due to poor socioeconomic conditions.
Marjolin's ulcer	Ulcer seated upon old cicatrix which follows the raking down of wart tumour.
McBurney's point	Pressure at this point (the point midway between the right anterior iliac spine and the umbilicus) elicits pain which is diagnostic of appendicitis.
Measles	An acute infectious disease caused by virus.
Meningitis	Infection and inflammation of the thin covering of brain and spinal cord.
Menorrhagia	Excessive flow of menstrual flow.
Metabolism	It is the combination of anabolism and catabolism in the body.
Midwifery	An art of attending to pregnant women in her pregnancy, in her delivery and in her post delivery period.
Migraine	Severe headache associated with nausea, vomiting and visual disturbances.
Miscarriage	Labour occurring before the 28th week of pregnancy.
Mountain Sickness	When a person is taken to high altitude he experiences certain clinical manifestations.
Mumps	A viral infection of parotid gland.
Myalgia	Pain experienced in muscle.
Myiasis	Breeding of larvae of common housefly in wounds.
Myxoedema	Hypothyroidism.

Napkin rash	Skin rash in infants in napkin area due to ammoniacal dermatitis.
Nephritis	Inflammation of kidney secondary to infection.
Night blindness	Vision problem during night which is associated with deficiency of vitamin A.
Nurse	Professional and qualified health personnel who is trained in nursing skills and nursing care; a trained person capable of performing nursing services under doctor's supervision.
Obesity	Overweight of a person which is more than 15% above normal weight or BMI of over 25 kg. per square metre of the body
Obstetrics	The discipline that deals with pregnancy, labour and puerperium.
Oedema	Fluid collection as a result of inflammatory process.
Open heart surgery	Surgery done on heart along with usage of cardiopulmonary heart lung machine.
Ophthalmia neonatorum	Severe purulent conjunctivitis of newborn by gonococci.
Opisthotonos	Body bending backwards seen in Tetanus
Orchitis	Infection and inflammation of testis.
Orgasm	Intense pleasure of sexual intercourse at climax.
ORS	Oral rehydration solution given for moderate dehydration.
Oxygen mask	Face mask for oxygen therapy to patient.
PUO	Pyrexia of Unknown Origin (fever where cause is not known).
Pain	It describes agony, intolerance, suffering and distress feeling.
Palsy	The term denotes paralysis which is associated with trembling and shaking.

Paralysis	Where there is loss of nervous function leading to loss of motion.
Paralytic ileus	When nurse auscultate abdomen bowel sounds are absent indicating emergency.
Para medical workers	Associated health workers who are trained in their skilled profession to help the doctor.
Parasite	Which live on another to fetch nourishment and thrive.
Para typhoid	Mild typhoid by mild strain typhoid bacteria.
Parkinson's disease	In extra pyramidal system, nuclear masses undergo degeneration giving rise to tremor, slow voluntary movements, festinating gait and peculiar posture.
Parotitis	Infection of parotid gland.
Pasteurisation	Heating of milk to kill pathogens.
Pelvimetry	Pelvic brim assessment for normal delivery.
Peristalsis	Wave like motion of stomach and intestine.
Peritonitis	Infection and inflammation of peritoneum.
Pertussis	Whooping cough.
Phimosis	Prepuce cannot be drawn back over glans penis.
Pigeon chest	Prominent sternum among children suffering from rickets.
Pimple	Papule or pustule on the face attributed to hormonal disturbances.
Pityriasis	Scaly desquamation of skin a known skin disorder.
Pneumoconiosis	Inhalation of dust produces chronic fibrous reaction in lung.
Pneumoperitoneum	Air is present in the peritoneal cavity.
Poliomyelitis	Acute viral infection that cause lameness, paralysis or death.

Polyp	Abnormal growth from a mucous membrane usually not malignant.
Pott's disease	Tuberculosis of spine.
Pregnancy	It starts with conception and implantation of fertilised ovum to delivery which is about 280 days.
Primary Health Care	It is "Essential health care based on practical, scientifically sound and socially acceptable methods and technology made universally accessible to individuals and families in the community through their full participation and at a cost that the community can afford to maintain at every state of their development in the spirit of self determination".
Primary Health Centre	It provides integrated health services to a specified population.
Psychosis	One of the specific mental illnesses.
Pterygium	Patch of thickened conjunctiva which extends even to cornea.
Pulse Polio immunisation	OPV is given to all 0 to 5 years children in a country on a single day regardless of previous immunisation.
Pyoderma	Skin disease with pus discharge.
Q fever	Rickettisial infection.
Quickening	Feeling of foetal movement by the mother during pregnancy
Quinsy	Peritonsillar abscess; an acute infection of tonsil.
Rabies	Hydrophobia by the bite of dog which has rabies virus in its saliva.
Rape	Sexual intercourse without consent.
Rash	Skin eruption due to infections or allergy.
Raynaud's disease	Cyanosis of fingers or toes on exposure to cold.
Resuscitation	Restoration of lung or heart function of a person.
Retrovirus	Which causes HIV/AIDS.
Rh factor	Rhesus factor. If mother is Rh-ve and newborn is Rh+ anaemia and jaundice

	occurs which is called Rh incompatibility.
Rheumatic fever	Acute infection of throat that can cause heart problem.
Rhinitis	Infection and inflammation of mucous membrane of the nose.
Ringer's solution	It is a type of IV fluid to rehydrate a person.
Ryle's tube	Used for withdrawal of gastric contents and used for administration of fluids.
Salpingitis	Fallopian tube infection.
Scabies	Skin condition produced by the itch mite.
Scurvy	Clinical condition due to vitamin C deficiency.
Senile	Loss of mental and emotional capacity
dementia	through physical changes in the brain as a result of hardening of the arteries in the brain.
Sequestrum	Necrosed bony part called dead bone in a living bone.
Shock treatment	Treatment of psychiatric patients by passing low voltage current.
SIFT	Semen intra fallopian tube transfer for infertility.
Sinusitis	Infection and inflammation of sinus like frontal sinus.
Skeleton	Supporting system of the body or bony framework.
Sleeping sickness	Trypanosoma infection transmitted by tsetse fly.
Small family norm	A concept to stabilise the population with 2 children per family which help to achieve NRR 1.0 and made acceptable to the lifestyle of people.
Snellen's chart	Sight testing chart.
Somnambulism	Carrying out activities during sleep.
Sore throat	Infection and inflammation of larynx, pharynx and tonsil.

Sphygmomanometer BP apparatus.

Squint Deviated eye which looks abnormal, turned inwards or outwards are common which are called convergent squint and divergent squint respectively.

Stenosis Pathological narrowing.

Stent Steel or plastic device kept in a vessel to keep it patent.

Strangulated Compressed and constricted hernia.

Strapping Application of strips of adhesive plaster.

Stroke Brain paralysis due to brain haemorrhage.

Surrogate mother Rent a womb to infertile couple constitutes surrogate motherhood.

Suture Surgical closure of a wound by catgut suture.

Tanning Skin changes produced by exposure to sunlight.

Tattoo Natural or chemical used in skin tattooing to produce permanent discolouration or a shaped picture.

Tennis elbow Occupational disorder where painful disorder develops in extensor muscle at elbow region.

Tenosynovitis Infection and inflammation of tendon and synovial sheath.

Tension headache Sustained contraction of muscles of head and neck cause tension headache.

Terminal care Care given to a patient in whom an incurable disease is present.

Tetanus Lock jaw or hydrophobia caused by a bacterial infection.

Thalassaemia Inheritance of abnormal haemoglobin causes haemolysis.

Thrush Vulvovaginal condition or balanitis by Candida fungal infection contracted through sexual activity.

Tinnitus Ringing in the ear.

Tracheostomy	Surgical opening in 4th tracheal cartilage for the purpose of artificial respiration, a life saving procedure.
Transplanta-tion	Process of transplant, replacement of failed organ with a healthy organ donated by another healthy person.
Travel sickness	Sea sickness common complaint of travellers who experience vomiting and nausea.
Trench foot	Effect of cold on feet due to ice, wet socks or wet shoes over a long period.
Tubectomy	Female sterilisation as permanent method of sterilisation.
Typhoid	Enteric infection spread through water.
Uraemia	It indicates the presence of urinary constituents in the blood.
UIP	Universal Immunisation Programme where infants are protected against 6 diseases and pregnant women are protected against tetanus.
Universal precaution	Procedure to protect oneself through precautions on universal blood and body fluid with all patients and at all time, which is also a measure to protect HIV/AIDS.
Uraemia	A disease state due to accumulation of wastes in the blood and tissues consequent upon kidney failure.
Urethritis	Infection and inflammation of urine discharging canal.
USG	Ultra sound lab investigation.
Vaginismus	Painful spasm of muscles of vagina during intercourse.
Vaginitis	Infection of female genital tract.
Venipuncture	Performing a puncture of a vein is necessary for administering IV fluids and medications.
Vertigo	Feeling of rotation of head in space even while at rest.
Viscera	An organ in the cavity of abdomen.

Ward management	Management of sick through medical and nursing care in the ward.
Warts	A virus infection of skin.
Wry neck	Neck torsion due to contraction of cervical muscles.
Xyster	File maintained by the surgeon.
Yellow fever	A viral infection, not present in India which is transmitted by mosquito.
Zidovudine	Drug used in HIV/AIDS.
Zoonoses	Disease of animal which man gets accidentally.

Chapter 10 Nursing Procedures' Terminology

Amniocentesis Drawing amniotic fluid through abdominal wall.

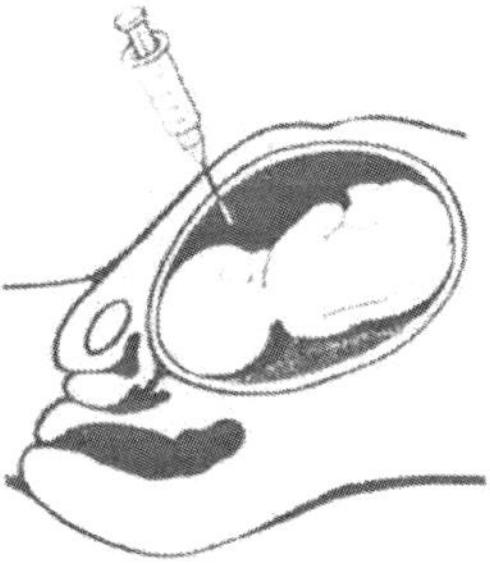

Fig 10.1: Amniocentesis

Amputation stump dressing Many tailed bandage is used in special dressing in case of amputation stump

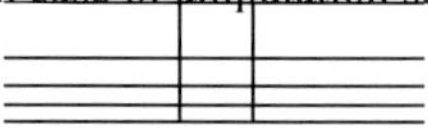

Many tailed

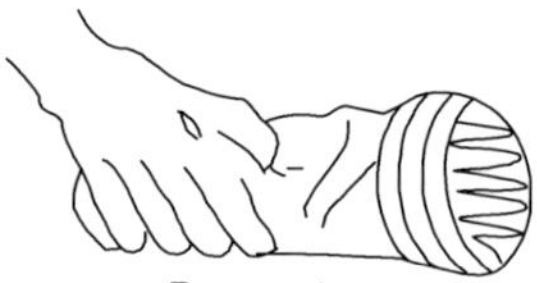

Recurrent

Fig. 10.2: Many tailed bandage for amputation stump and recurrent bandage for amputation stump

Ankle exercise Part of exercise in nursing care to assist patient in positioning and mobilisation.

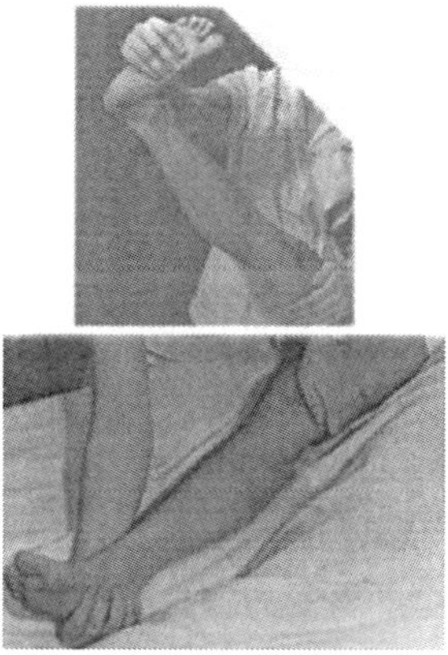

Fig. 10.3: Ankle exercise

Apgar score A system of newborn assessment.

Aspiration of chest Removing a collection of fluid from the pleural cavity.

Auditory assessment Assessing auditory function by watch test or Weber and Rinne's Tuning fork tost.

Autolet An automatic device for blood glucose testing in diabetes.

Ballottement A test used in pregnancy, abdominal palpation of uterus, in PV exami-nation a finger push upwards rebounds back.

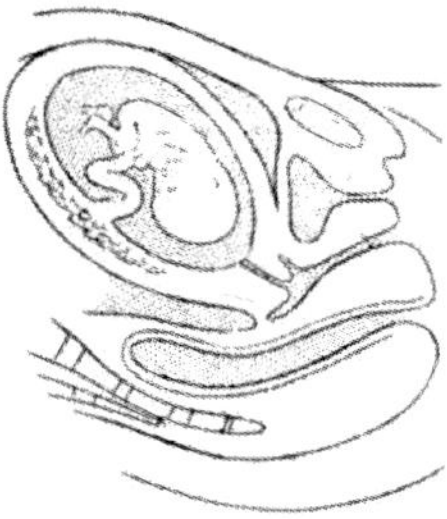

Fig. 10.4: Ballottement

Bladder irrigation Done for cystitis, include catheterisation and irrigation of bladder.

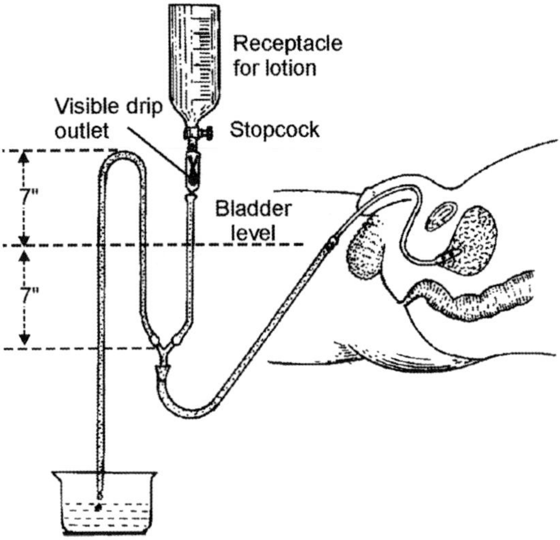

Fig. 10.5: Bladder irrigation

Bellows resuscitator A modified bag used to produce positive pressure ventilation as an alternative to the first aiders own breath.

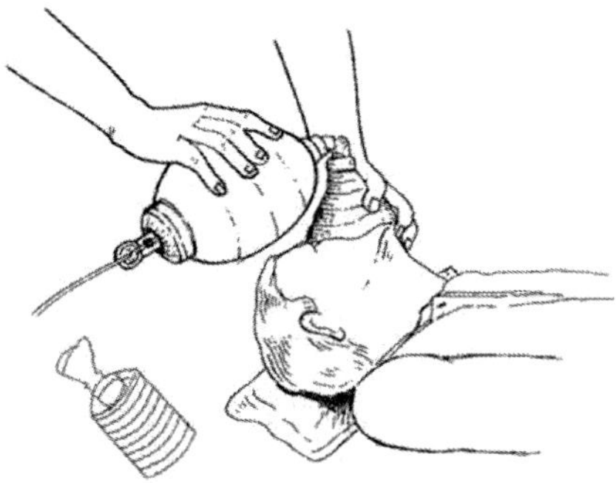

Fig. 10.6: Bellow in Ambu resuscitator

B.P. recording Assessing systolic and diastolic blood pressure.

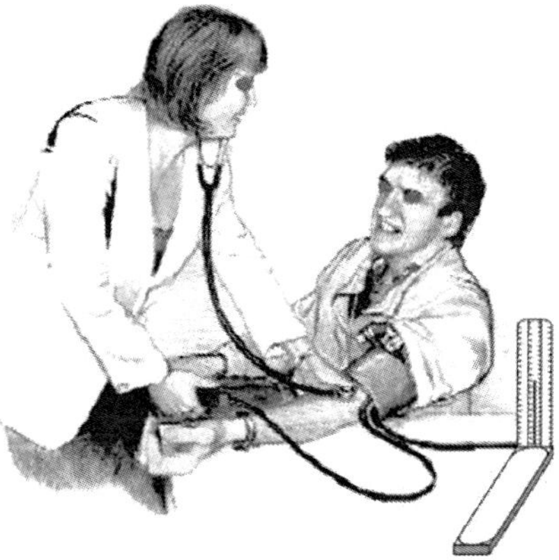

Fig.10.7: BP recording

Bulb syringe Normal item kept in newborn's crib for removing secretions in the nose and mouth.

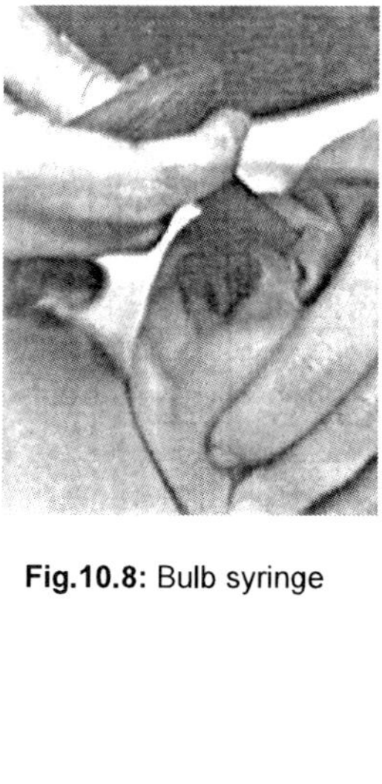

Fig.10.8: Bulb syringe

Chest bandage First aid measure in chest injury.

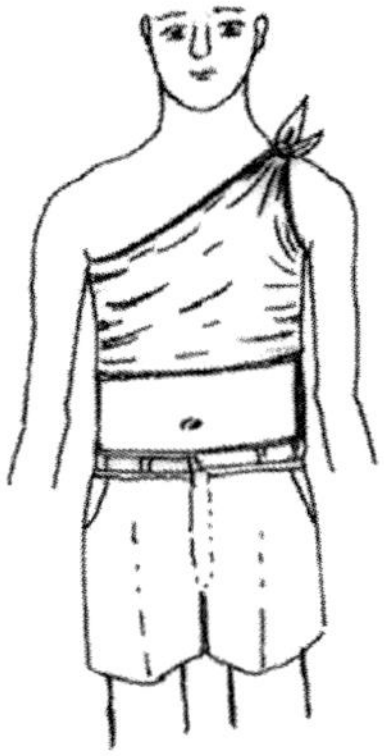

Fig. 10.9: Chest bandage

Cradle hold Commonly used position for breast-feeding in which mother is sitting upright, with the infant's head held in the crook of her arm and its buttocks cradled in her hand. Nurse has to teach this.

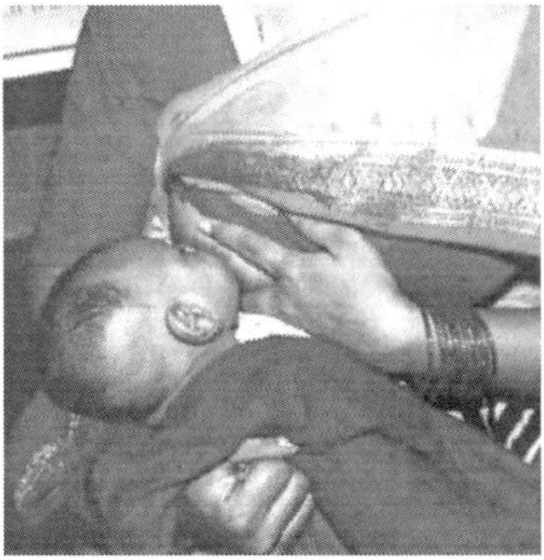

Fig.10.10: Cradle hold

D & C OBG procedure done for diagnosis and therapy. Dilatation and curettage.

Enema Enema is an injection of fluid into the rectum and this is ordered for the following reasons:

- To empty the bowel of faeces.
- To relieve distension due to flatus.
- To introduce drugs or fluids.
- For diagnostic purpose.

Episiotomy Surgical incision done during second stage of labour to facilitate childbirth in primi gravida, this helps to avoid damage to perineal muscles during childbirth.

Examination of lower lid It is done to find out redness, congestion, watering, foreign body or any ulcer.

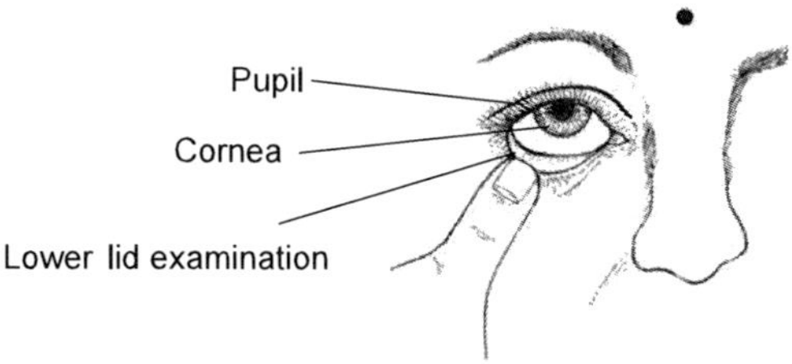

Fig.10.11: Examination of lower lid

Eyedrops Medicamentation to the eye in case of infection or inflammation put through dropper.

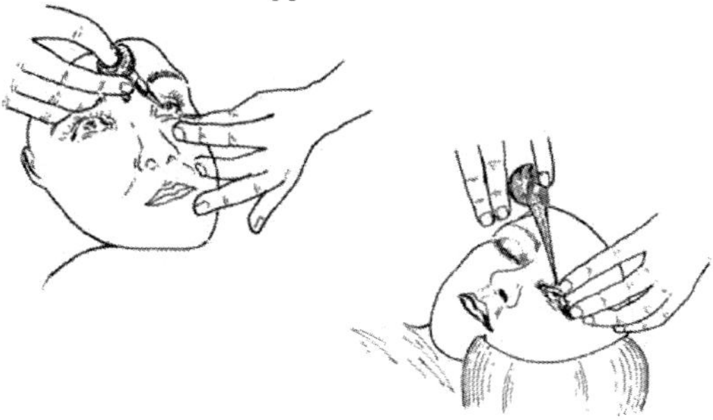

Fig. 10.12: Application of eyedrops and irrigation of eye

Fleets enema It is a type of retention enema.

Football hold This is recommended to mothers who have had a caesarean delivery because it enables them to support the infant's weight off their abdomen. Nurse should teach this.

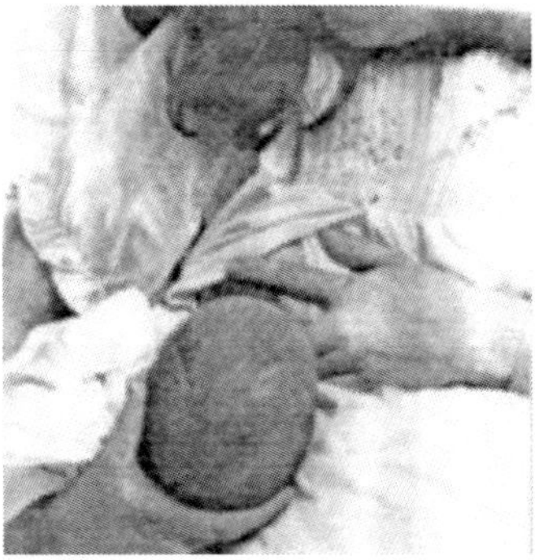

Fig. 10.13: Football hold

Gastric lavage Washing out the stomach is indicted in pyloric stenosis, intestinal obstruction immediately before operation and in the treatment for poisoning when a poison is swallowed.

Glasgow Coma Scale To monitor level of consciousness in adults this scale is used.

Group counselling It helps in realising family potential or group potential to help themselves in contrast to helping them.

Growth chart They are used for recording weight of children corresponding to their given age.

Gynaecologic technique Performing routine gynaecologic techniques refers to the examination of the following female reproductive system:

- Breast examination.
- Breast self-examination.

- Post mastectomy exercises.
- Providing perineal care.
- Cervical uterine radiation implant.

Gynaecological examination A nurse should learn the preparation of patient for gynaecological examination for:
- PV examination.
- Douching.
- Vulval toilet.
- Vaginal pessary.

Hand rolls Used for flaccid patients in spinal injuries.

Heimlich manoeuvre It is an emergency manoeuvre for foreign body in trachea.

Holdger Nielsen Resuscitation Introduced in Denmark, used by Red Cross. Essential movements of pressing and arm rising not only ventilate the lungs but also stimulate the heart.

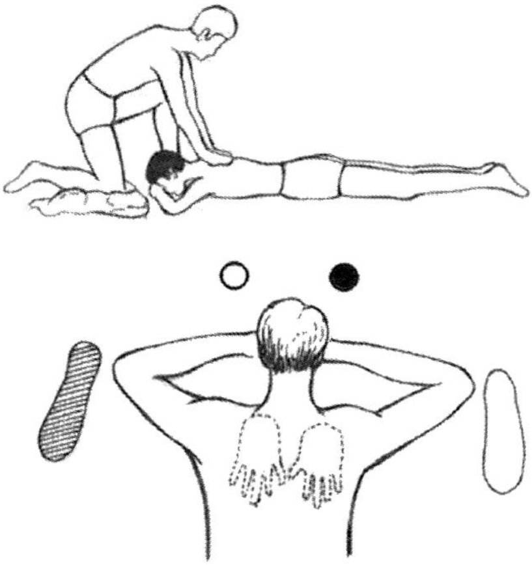

Fig.10.14

Home care instructions This is the instructions to mother for the care of her newborn or her child.

Indwelling catheter Performing a catheterisation with a Foley catheter.

Injections Giving medicaments to a person by route other than mouth like subcunataneous injection, intradermal injection, intravenous injection, hypodermic injection, depot injection, intrathecal injection.

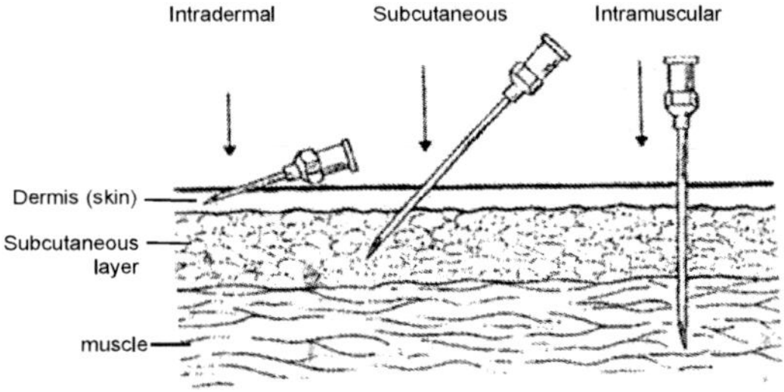

Fig. 10.15: Routes of injections

Intravenous Method of giving drug or medicamentaion through vein, emergency medication method. Method of giving nutrition to patients.

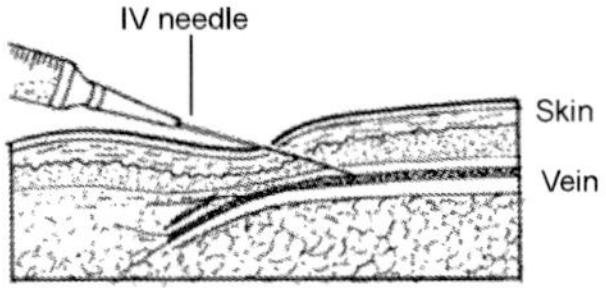

Fig.10.16: IV needle in position

Kidney palpation A comprehensive assessment by palpation of kidney to assess for difference in size, absence of kidney, mass, nodule and for the discomfort.

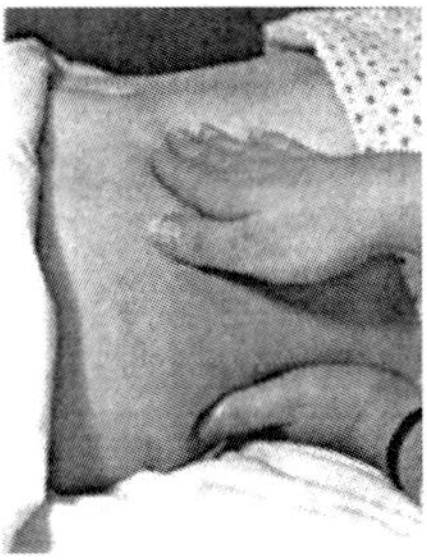

Fig. 10.17: Palpating the kidney

Leopold's maneuvers This is performed to determine foetal position, hands at examination is made warmer and maneuver is done in-between uterine contractions which can either be labour contractions or Broxton Hicks contractions.

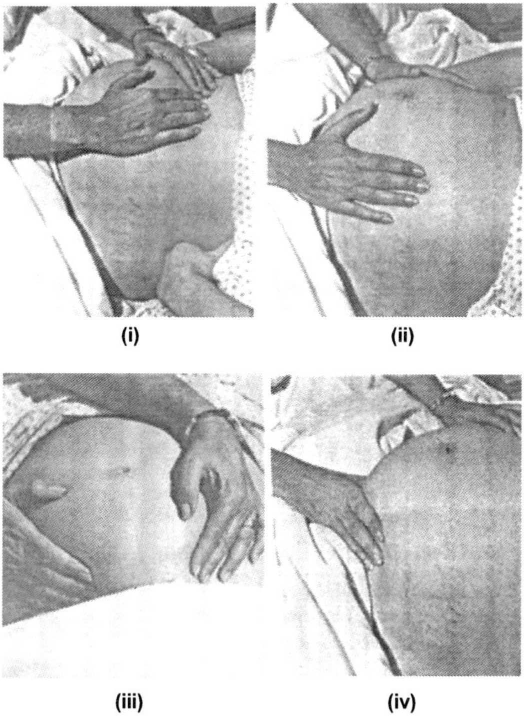

Fig. 10.18: (i) First maneuver, (ii) Second maneuver, (iii) Third maneuver, and (iv) Fourth maneuver

Lithotomy position This is common position for gynaecological examination.

Log rolling It is done to the immobile patients; if patient has a neck injury or a spinal disorder, it will be necessary for the nurse to log roll the patient.

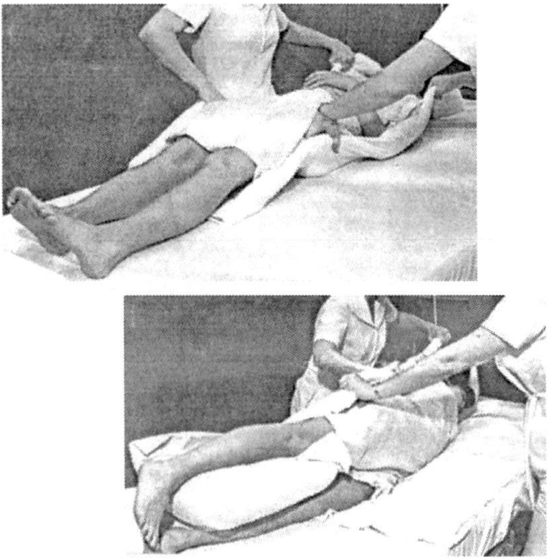

Fig. 10.19A and B: Log rolling the patient

Making oral fluid For mild dehydration this is prepared which is called ORS.

Oesophageal feeding It is tube feeding to describe the administration of fluid food through a tube passed into the stomach either through mouth or through nose, they are done under doctor's order. This requires another nurse assistance.

Oxygen therapy It is an utmost requirement of managing respiration therapy.

Paracentesis It is tapping the abdomen to draw fluid from peritoneal cavity particularly in liver disorder and malignancy.

Perineal care This is routine gynaecological technique done and or supervised by the nurse.

Pessaries It is an instrument for introduction into the vagina for giving support in case of prolapse uterus. Nurse usually introduces ring pessary.

Phototherapy Premature infants experience jaundice because of increased serum bilirubin level. Phototherapy is given to overcome hyperbilirubinaemia. Entire skin of infant is exposed to light for given period of time.

Piggyback medication Through an established IV set, medication is given by a secondary bottle called piggyback bottle.

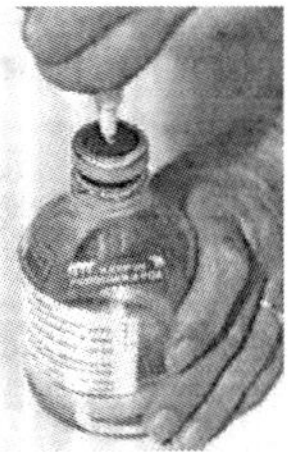

Fig. 10.20: Piggyback infusion bottle ready for attachment

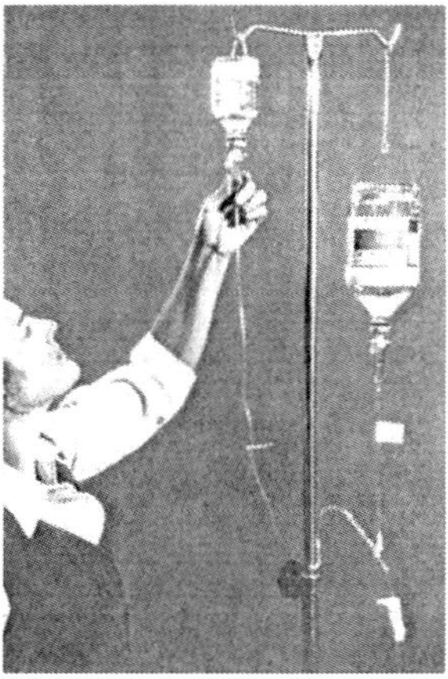

Fig. 10.21: Piggyback bottle is fixed to the established IV set

Positioning aids To prevent abnormal movements of parts of the body positioning aids are given, like Trochanter rolls, sandbags, foot supports and hand rolls.

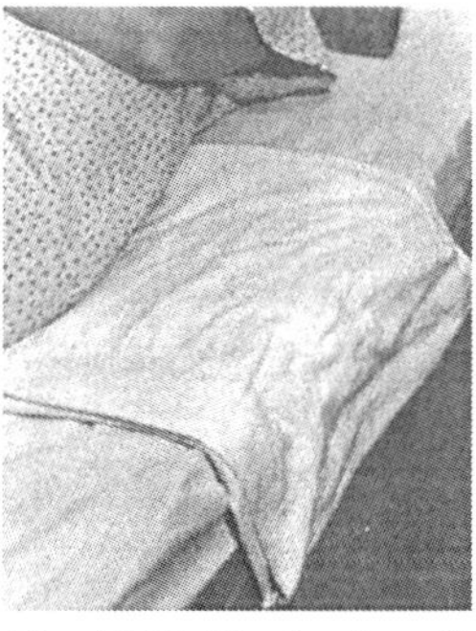

Fig. 10.22: Trochanter roll is being started at bed

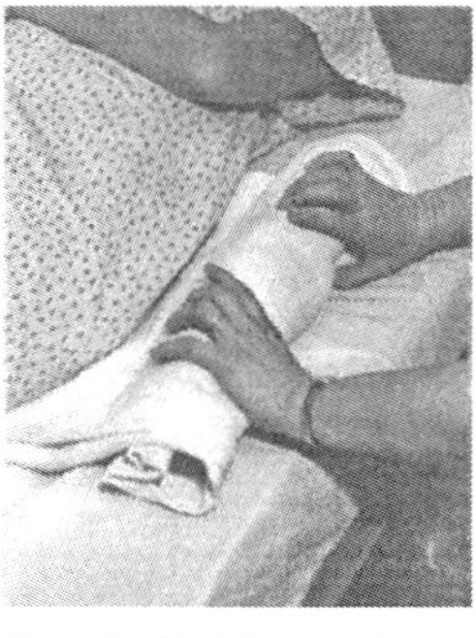

Fig. 10.23: Trochanter roll ready to tuck against patients hip

Presumptive treatment All fever cases are given malaria treatment presuming fever could be by malaria.

Radical treatment All malaria smear positive cases are given one course of radical treatment for malaria.

Rectal examination Before PR examination, privacy is provided, procedure is explained and patient is put in Sim's position, inspected for piles, skin changes, cysts and fissures.

Residual limb wrapping Post operatively a residual limb is wrapped with elastic bandage to reduce swelling and to mould the stump for eventual prosthetic fitting.

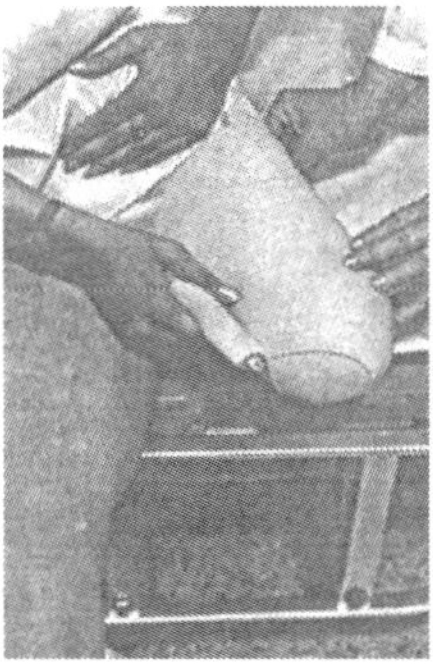

Fig. 10.24: Residual limb wrapping

Taping IV needle Use of 3 inches strips of tape for fixing the IV needle introduced in IV therapy.

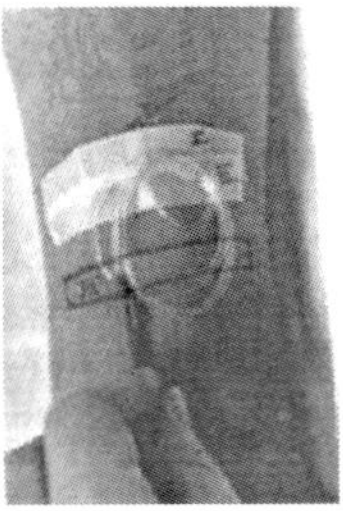

Fig.10.25: Taping (to tape the needle) the needle for IV therapy

Tracheostomy cuff Used to maintain patent airway in emergency case management.

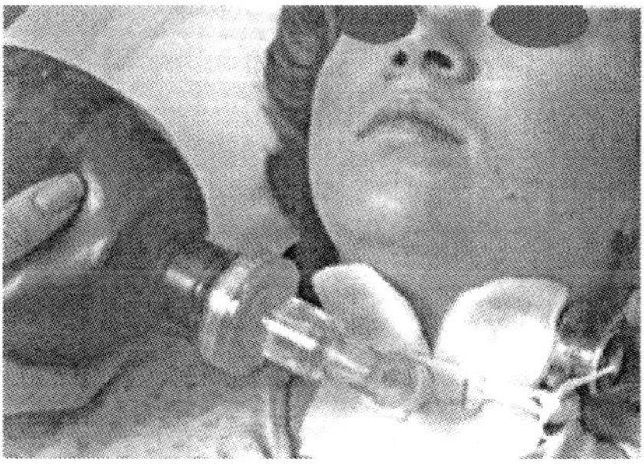

Fig.10.26: Managing tracheostomy cuffs

Trochanter rolls To prevent abduction and external rotation of hip, a bath blanket which is folded and positioned from waist to mid thigh for draping.

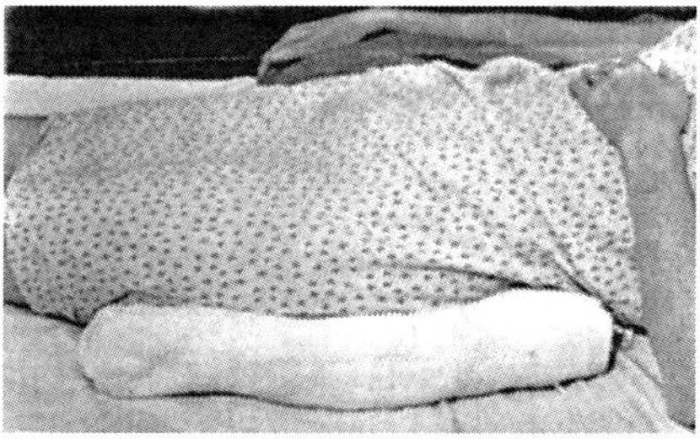

Fig.10.27: Positioning aid by trochanter roll

Tuberculin test A skin test which shows whether or not an individual has received tuberculus bacilli in his body.

Vacutainer Collecting the blood sample with a vacuum container. Vacuum container is vacutainer.

Vaginal douching Done for cleansing purpose in cases of vaginal discharge, preoperative, when vaginal pessary is used.

Vaginal examination	Done for diagnosis, smear taking, pre-operative, dorsal or lithotomy position are used.
Vaginal irrigation	Douche, indicated in preoperative cleansing with povidone iodine solution.
Venipuncture	Performing a puncture of a vein is necessary for administering IV fluid and medications.

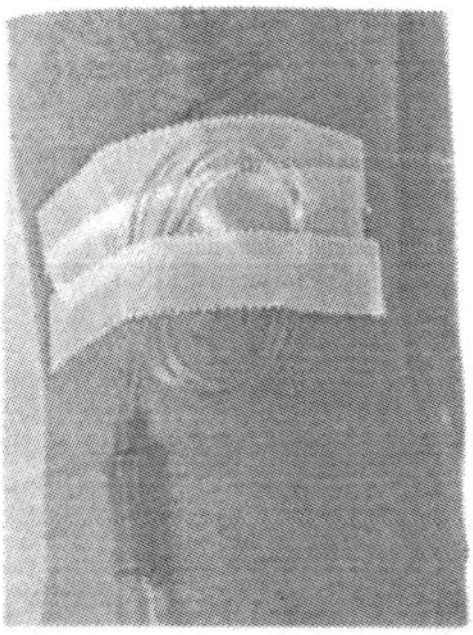

Fig. 10.28: Venipuncture

Wet to dry dressing	Refers to packing a wound either with medication or without medication.
Z tract injection	When Iron injection is to be given to gluteal region. 2 Track is followed.

Chapter 11 Phonetics

PHONETICS IN ENGLISH

The word 'Phonetics' is from Greek meaning the **study of sound produced** in our voice or in our speech. Phonetics deals with the English sounds themselves rather than context of their usage. Phoneticians are more concerned with sounds of speech than symbols. Part of phonetics is semiotics which is the study of symbols.

Phonetics are 3 types:

1. Articulatory - Involving position and movement of lips, tongue, vocal folds.
2. Acoustic - Involve property of sound waves and how received by ear.
3. Auditory - Involved in speech perception i.e., how brain receives.

English language has:

13 vowel phonemes.

24 consonant phonemes.

Historically Tamil grammar book *Tolkappiyam* (5th century BC) and Sanskrit grammar described many of articulations.

English is a global language spoken by 350 million people as I language, 280 million as II language across 104 countries.

Pronunciations

The sounds represented are as per British English spoken Pronunciation accent.

English alphabets

Aa	Bb	Cc	Dd	Ee	Ff	Gg	Hh
[eɪ]	[bi:]	[sɪ:]	[di:]	[i:]	[ɛf]	[dʒi:]	[eɪtʃ]
Ii	**Jj**	**Kk**	**Ll**	**Mm**	**Nn**	**Oo**	**Pp**
[aɪ]	[dʒeɪ]	[keɪ]	[ɛl]	[ɛm]	[ɛn]	[əʃ]	[pi:]
Qq	**Rr**	**Ss**	**Tt**	**Uu**	**Vv**	**Ww**	**Xx**
[kju:]	[ɑ:]	[ɛs]	[ti:]	[ju:]	[vi:]	['dʃbəlju:]	[ɛks]
Yy	**Zz**						
[waɪ]	[zɛd/zi:]						

Vowels

ɑ: father ['fɑ:ðə], **alms** [ɑ:ms], **clerk** [klɑ:k], **heart** [hɑ:t], sergeant [sɑ:dʒənt]

ɒ pot [pɒt], botch [bɒtʃ], sorry ['sɒrɪ]

æ cat [kæt], plait [plæt]

ɛ bet [bɛt], ate [ɛt], bury ['bɛrɪ], heifer ['hɛfa], said [sɛd], says [sɛz]

ə potter ['pɒtə], alone [ə'lə ʃn], furious [fjʃ ərɪəs], nation [neɪʃən], the [ðə]

ɜ: fern [fɜ:n], burn [bɜ:n], fir [fɜ:], learn [lɜ:n], term [tɜ:m], worm [wɜ:m]

ɪ pretty ['prɪtɪ] build [bɪld], busy ['bɪzɪ], nymph [nɪmf], pocket ['pɒkɪt], sieve [sɪv], women ['wɪmɪn]

i: see [si:], aesthete ['i:sθi:t], evil ['i: vəl], magazine [ˌmæga'zi:n], receive [rɪ'si:v], siege [si:dʒ]

ɔ thaw [θɔ:], broad [brɔ:d], drawer ['drɔ:ə], fault [fɔ:lt], halt [hɔ:lt], organ ['ɔ:gən]

ʃ pull [pʃ l], good [gʃ d], should [ʃ ʃd], woman ['wʃ mən]

u: zoo [zu:], do [du:], queue [kju:], shoe [ʃu:], spew [spju:], true [tru:], you [ju:]

ʃ cut [kʃ t], flood [flʃ d], rough [rʃ f], son [sʃ n]

Diphthongs

aɪ dive [daɪv], aisle [aɪl], guy [gaɪ], might [maɪt], rye [raɪ]

aɪə fire ['faɪə], buyer ['baɪə], liar ['laɪə], tyre ['taɪə]

aʃ out [aʃ t], bough [baʃ], crowd [kraʃ d], slouch [slaʃ tʃ]

aʃ ə flour ['flaʃ ə], cower ['caʃ ə], flower ['flaʃ ə], sour ['saʃ ə]

eɪ paid [peɪd], day [deɪ], deign [deɪn], gauge [geɪdʒ], grey [greɪ], neigh [neɪ]

ɛə bear [bɛə], dare [bɛə], prayer [prɛə], stairs [stɛəz], where [wɛə]

ɪə tear [tɪə], beer [bɪə], mere [mɪə], tier [tɪə]

əʃ note [nəʃ t], beau [bəʃ], dough [dəʃ], hoe [həʃ], slow [sləʃ], yeoman ['jəʃ mən]

ɔɪ void [vɔɪd], boy [bɔɪ], destroy [dɪ'strɔɪ]

ʃə poor [pʃ ə], skewer ['skjʃ ə], sure [fʃ ə]

Consonants

p pig [pɪg], **b** big [bɪg], **t** tea [tɪ:], **d** dactylology [ˌdæktɪ' lɒlədʒɪ]

k kangaroo [ˌkæŋga'ru:], cacophony [kə'kɒfani]

g get [gɛt], ghoul [gu:l], guard [ga:d], examine [ɪ'gzæmɪn]

m **mamm**oth ['mæməθ]
n **n**yctophobia [ˌnɪktəʃ faʃ bɪe], **kn**owledge ['nɒlɪdʒ], **gn**otobiotics [ˌnəʃ təʃ baɪ'ɒtɪks], **pn**eumatic ['njʃ mætɪk]
ŋ si**ng** [siŋ], phary**n**x ['færɪŋks]
r **r**adio ['reɪdɪəʃ], **rh**inoceros [raɪ'nɒsərəs / raɪ'nɒsrəs]
f **f**oxtrot ['fɒksˌtrɒt], **ph**oenix ['fi:nɪks], **v** **v**arious ['vεərɪəs]
θ **th**in [θin], **ð** **th**ese [ði:z]
s **s**illy ['sɪlɪ], **c**ircus ['sɜ: kəs]
z **z**ebra ['zi:brə / 'zebrə], **x**ero**x** ['zɪərɒks]
ʃ **sh**ip [ʃɪp], elec**ti**on [ɪ'lεkʃən], ma**ch**ine [mə'ʃi:n], mi**ssi**on ['mɪʃən], pre**ss**ure ['prεʃə], **sch**edule ['ʃεdju:l]
ʒ trea**s**ure ['trεʒə], a**z**ure ['æʒə], eva**si**on [ɪ'vəiʒən]
h **h**otel [həʃ 'tεl]
l **l**atera**l** ['lætərəl]
j **y**es [jεs], on**i**on [' ʃnjən], vi**gn**ette [vi'njεt]
tʃ **ch**ew [tʃu:] na**t**ure ['neɪtʃə]
dʒ **j**aw [dʒɔ:] a**dj**ective ['ædʒɪktɪv], sol**di**er ['səʃ ldʒe], usa**ge** ['ju:sɪdʒ]
w **w**et [wεt], **wh**eel [wi:l]

Vowels

Long vowels		*Short vowels*			
i:	sheep	ɪ	ship	e	head
ɑ:	farm	æ	hat	ə	above
u:	coo	ʃ	foot	ɚ	mother (US)
ɔ:	horse	ɒ	sock (UK)		
ɜ:	bird	ʃ	cup		

Consonants

b	book	p	pen
d	day	t	town
g	give	k	cat
v	very	f	fish
ð	the	θ	think
z	zoo	s	say
ʒ	vision	ʃ	she
dʒ	jump	tʃ	cheese
l	look		
r	run		
j	yes		
w	we		
m	moon		
n	name		
ŋ	sing		

Diphthongs

eɪ	day
aɪ	eye
ɔɪ	boy
aʃ	mouth
eʃ	nose (UK)
oʃ	nose (US)

ɪə ear (UK)
eə hair (UK)
ʃə pure (UK)

Other symbols

h	hand	
ɔ̃:	/'res.tər.ɔ̃:/	restaurant
i	/'hæp.i/	happy
ţ	/'bʃţ.ɚ/	butter (US)
u	/ˌɪn.flu'en.zə/	influenza
l̩	/'lɪt.l̩/	little

əl əm ən can be pronounced either /əl/ or /l̩/ etc.
/'leɪ.bəl/ → /'leɪ.bəl /or /'leɪ.bl̩/ label

r	linking r is pronounced only before a vowel in British English: /fɔ:r/ → /fɔ:ræp.l̩z/ four → four apples	
ˈ	main stress	/ˌek.spek'teɪ.ʃən/ expectation
ˌ	secondary stress	/ˌri:'tel/ retell
.	syllable division	/'sɪs.təm/

Chapter 12

Public Speech

Public speech has been an armamentarium of Politicians, Leaders and Religious Heads since centuries. Public speeches are recorded and accorded as memorable ones in kingly provinces.

Dr. S. Radhakrishnan, Mr.Winston Churchill, John F Kennedy, Elisabeth I, Martin Luther King have achieved prominence in public life because they were effective speakers.

All said and done all eminent people have shown their own method of becoming prominent as Public Speakers. All had two things in common. They were:

—careful preparation of speeches.

—careful presentation of speeches.

The Public Speech is defined as under:

"It is speaking in public gathering, fluently without interruption, focussing sharply toward public interest and public attitude, which can be an art to rule the minds of public."

"Well prepared, well outlined, well delivered in an effective manner and clearing any doubts in the minds of public constitute Public Speech."

Preparation for a Public Speech

When you are giving a public speech, get to know what is expected of you by the public. To focus your speech towards public interest gets to know the type of gathering. Age, gender and occupation of such public can demand their own requirement.

Think of possible arguments and about your conclusion in public speech. Time management is important. Gather your material for preparing an outline of your public speech.

Developing an Outline of Public Speech

Structuring the public speech by following steps of principles:

No. 1	Follow the speech topic by topic.
No. 2	Make your speech suitable to the area of speech.
No. 3	Make the theme chronological and by updated information.
No. 4	Take problems and sort out solutions.

Delivering the Speech in an Effective Manner

Clear outline, well judged content allow effective delivery of speech.

Impromptu speech is not advisable. It is okay if public speech is given by meamorising content and structure in the mind.

Using notes or points comes next.

Third one is reading the script which is ineffective.

You can adopt Winston Churchill method of marking *pause, louder* etc., which is combined with gestures.

Always look at the audience during your speech.

Before giving speech, trying on friends, colleagues or relatives is best advocated.

Short sentences and simple language are highly appreciable.

Well-known speakers like John F Kennedy have adopted Rhetorical tricks to get key points through **repetition**, **contrast** and **lists of three**.

Gestures are appreciated.

Speaking at Social Events

The same effective manner can be adopted in speaking at social events like:

- Welcoming a visitor.
- Presenting an award.
- Farewell speeches.

- proposing a toast.
- Replying to a toast.
- Accepting an award.

Equip Oneself for Public Speech

Before your public speech, check all equipment you need. Check whether they work. Get to know how they work. It can be Microphone clip on radio microphone is better as they allow freedom of movement.

Check if you can see everybody and they can also see you.

To Take off Stage Fear

Nervousness with adrenaline pumping madly in the body can paralyse the speech in a public speech. When controlled, it can lift the performance.

Public Speech and Public Interaction

Develop the habit of eliciting questions from audience and answer them. In the beginning you can announce the question time at the end. Audience will prepare and ask you questions.

Differentiate between Questions and Suggestions.

FAMOUS PUBLIC SPEECHES

Speech 01

Swami Vivekananda Speech

Chicago, Sept 11, 1893

Sisters and Brothers of America

It fills my heart with joy unspeakable to rise in response to the warm and cordial welcome which you have given us. I thank you in the name of the most ancient order of monks in the world; I thank you in the name of the mother of religions, and I thank you in the name of millions and millions of Hindu people of all classes and sects.

My thanks, also, to some of the speakers on this platform who, referring to the delegates from the Orient, have told you that these men from far-off nations may well claim the honor of bearing to different lands the idea of toleration. I am proud to belong to a religion which has taught the world both tolerance and universal acceptance. We believe not only in universal toleration, but we accept all religions as true. I am proud to belong to a nation which has sheltered the persecuted and the refugees of all religions and all nations of the earth. I am proud to tell you that we have gathered in our bosom the purest remnant of the Israelites, who came to Southern India and took refuge with us in the very year in which their holy temple was shattered to pieces by Roman tyranny. I am proud to belong to the religion which has sheltered and is still fostering the remnant of the grand Zoroastrian nation. I will quote to you, brethren, a few lines from a hymn which I remember to have repeated from my earliest boyhood, which is every day repeated by millions of human beings: "As the different streams having their sources in different paths which men take through different tendencies, various though they appear, crooked or straight, all lead to Thee."

The present convention, which is one of the most august assemblies ever held, is in itself a vindication, a declaration to the world of the wonderful doctrine preached in the Gita: "Whosoever comes to Me, through whatsoever form, I reach him; all men are struggling through paths which in the end lead to me." Sectarianism, bigotry, and its horrible descendant, fanaticism, have long possessed this beautiful earth. They have filled the earth with violence, drenched it often and often with human blood, destroyed civilization and sent whole nations to despair. Had it not been for these horrible demons, human society would be far more advanced than it is now. But their time is come; and I fervently hope that the bell that tolled this morning in honor of this convention may be the death-knell of all fanaticism, of all persecutions with the sword or with the pen, and of all uncharitable feelings between persons wending their way to the same goal.

Speech 02

Swamy Vivekananda Speech

Chicago, Sept 27, 1893

The World's Parliament of Religions has become an accomplished fact, and the merciful Father has helped those who laboured to bring it into existence, and crowned with success their most unselfish labour.

My thanks to those noble souls whose large hearts and love of truth first dreamed this wonderful dream and then realized it. My thanks to the shower of liberal sentiments that has overflowed this platform. My thanks to this enlightened audience for their uniform kindness to me and for their appreciation of every thought that tends to smooth the friction of religions. A few jarring notes were heard from time to time in this harmony. My special thanks to them, for they have, by their striking contrast, made general harmony the sweeter.

Much has been said of the common ground of religious unity. I am not going just now to venture my own theory. But if any one here hopes that this unity will come by the triumph of any one of the religions and the destruction of the others, to him I say, "Brother, yours is an impossible hope." Do I wish that the Christian would become Hindu? God forbid. Do I wish that the Hindu or Buddhist would become Christian? God forbid.

The seed is put in the ground, and earth and air and water are placed around it. Does the seed become the earth, or the air, or the water? No. It becomes a plant. It develops after the law of its own growth, assimilates the air, the earth, and the water, converts them into plant substance, and grows into a plant.

Similar is the case with religion. The Christian is not to become a Hindu or a Buddhist, nor a Hindu or a Buddhist to become a Christian. But each must assimilate the spirit of the others and yet preserve his individuality and grow according to his own law of growth.

If the Parliament of Religions has shown anything to the world, it is this: It has proved to the world that holiness, purity and charity are not the exclusive possessions of any church in the world, and that every system has produced men and women of the most exalted character. In the face of this evidence, if anybody dreams of the exclusive survival of his own religion and the destruction of the others, I pity him from the bottom of my heart, and point out to him that upon the banner of every religion will soon be written in spite of resistance: "Help and not fight", "Assimilation and not Destruction." "Harmony and Peace and not Dissension."

Speech 03

Speech by Abraham Lincoln

Gettysburg, Nov, 19, 1893

Four score and seven years ago our fathers brought forth on this continent a new nation, conceived in liberty and dedicated to the proposition that all men are created equal.

Now we are engaged in a great civil war, testing whether that nation or any nation so conceived and so dedicated can long endure. We are met on a great battlefield of that war.

We have come to dedicate a portion of that field as a final resting-place for those who here gave their lives that that nation might live. It is altogether fitting and proper that we should do this.

But in a larger sense, we cannot dedicate, we cannot consecrate, we cannot hallow this ground. The brave men, living and dead who struggled here have consecrated it far above our poor power to add or detract.

The world will little note nor long remember what we say here, but it can never forget what they did here. It is for us the living rather to be dedicated here to the unfinished work which they who fought here have thus far so nobly advanced.

It is rather for us to be here dedicated to the great task remaining before us—that from these honored dead we take increased devotion to that cause for which they gave the last full measure of devotion.

That we here highly resolve that these dead shall not have died in vain, that this nation under God shall have a new birth of freedom, and that government of the people, by the people, for the people shall not perish from the earth...

Speech 04

Speech of Winston Churchill

House of Commons, May 13, 1840

On Friday evening last I received from His Majesty the mission to form a new administration. It was the evident will of Parliament and the nation that this should be conceived on the broadest possible basis and that it should include all parties. I have already completed the most important part of this task.

A war cabinet has been formed of five members, representing, with the Labour, Opposition, and Liberals, the unity of the nation. It was necessary that this should be done in one single day on account of the extreme urgency and rigor of events. Other key positions were filled yesterday. I am submitting a further list to the king tonight. I hope to complete the appointment of principal ministers during tomorrow.

The appointment of other ministers usually takes a little longer. I trust when Parliament meets again this part of my task will be completed and that the administration will be complete in all respects. I considered it in the public interest to suggest to the Speaker that the House should be summoned today. At the end of today's proceedings, the adjournment of the House will be proposed until May 21 with provision for earlier meeting if need be. Business for that will be notified to MPs at the earliest opportunity.

I now invite the House by a resolution to record its approval of the steps taken and declare its confidence in the new government.

The Resolution:

"That this House welcomes the formation of a government representing the united and inflexible resolve of the nation to prosecute the war with Germany to a victorious conclusion."

To form an administration of this scale and complexity is a serious undertaking in itself. But we are in the preliminary phase of one of the greatest battles in history. We are in action at many other points-in Norway and in Holland-and we have to be prepared in the Mediterranean. The air battle is continuing, and many preparations have to be made here at home.

In this crisis I think I may be pardoned if I do not address the House at any length today, and I hope that any of my friends and colleagues or former colleagues who are affected by the political reconstruction will make all allowances for any lack of ceremony with which it has been necessary to act.

I say to the House as I said to ministers who have joined this government, I have nothing to offer but blood, toil, tears and sweat. We have before us an ordeal of the most grievous kind. We have before us many, many months of struggle and suffering.

You ask, what is our policy? I say it is to wage war by land, sea and air. War with all our might and with all the strength God has given us, and to wage war against a monstrous tyranny never surpassed in the dark and lamentable catalogue of human crime. That is our policy.

You ask, what is our aim? I can answer in one word. It is victory. Victory at all costs—Victory in spite of all terrors—Victory, however long and hard the road may be, for without victory there is no survival.

Let that be realized. No survival for the British Empire, no survival for all that the British Empire has stood for, no survival for the urge, the impulse of the ages, that mankind shall move forward toward his goal.

I take up my task in buoyancy and hope. I feel sure that our cause will not be suffered to fail among men. I feel entitled at this juncture, at this time, to claim the aid of all and to say, "Come then, let us go forward together with our united strength."

Speech 05

Speech of Martin Luther King

Aug. 28, 1963 at Lincoln Memorial in Washington DC

I am happy to join with you today in what will go down in history as the greatest demonstration for freedom in the history of our nation.

Five score years ago, a great American, in whose symbolic shadow we stand today, signed the Emancipation Proclamation. This momentous decree came as a great beacon light of hope to millions of Negro slaves who had been seared in the flames of withering injustice. It came as a joyous daybreak to end the long night of their captivity.

But one hundred years later, the Negro still is not free. One hundred years later, the life of the Negro is still sadly crippled by the manacles of segregation and the chains of discrimination. One hundred years later, the Negro lives on a lonely island of poverty in the midst of a vast ocean of material prosperity. One hundred years later, the Negro is still languished in the corners of American society and finds himself an exile in his own land. And so we've come here today to dramatize a shameful condition.

In a sense we've come to our nation's capital to cash a cheque. When the architects of our republic wrote the magnificent words of the Constitution and the Declaration of Independence, they were signing a promissory note to which every American was to fall heir. This note was a promise that all men, yes, black men as well as white men, would be guaranteed the "unalienable Rights" of "Life, Liberty and the pursuit of Happiness." It is obvious today that America has defaulted on this promissory note, insofar as her citizens of color are concerned. Instead of honoring this sacred obligation, America has given the Negro people a bad cheque, a cheque which has come back marked "insufficient funds".

But we refuse to believe that the bank of justice is bankrupt. We refuse to believe that there are insufficient funds in the great vaults of opportunity of this nation. And so, we've come to cash this cheque, a cheque that will give us upon demand the riches of freedom and the security of justice.

We have also come to this hallowed spot to remind America of the fierce urgency of Now. This is no time to engage in the luxury of cooling off or to take the tranquillizing drug of gradualism. Now is the time to make real the promises of democracy. Now is the time to rise from the dark and desolate valley of segregation to the sunlit path of racial justice. Now is the time to lift our nation from the quicksands of racial injustice to the solid rock of brotherhood. Now is the time to make justice a reality for all of God's children.

It would be fatal for the nation to overlook the urgency of the moment. This sweltering summer of the Negro's legitimate discontent will not pass until there is an invigorating autumn of freedom and equality. Nineteen-sixty-three is not an end, but a beginning. And those who hope that the Negro needed to blow off steam and will now be content will have a rude awakening if the nation returns to business as usual. And there will be neither rest nor tranquillity in America until the Negro is granted his citizenship rights. The whirlwinds of revolt will continue to shake the foundations of our nation until the bright day of justice emerges.

But there is something that I must say to my people, who stand on the warm threshold which leads into the palace of justice: In the process of gaining our rightful place, we must not be guilty of wrongful deeds. Let us not seek to satisfy our thirst for freedom by drinking from the cup of bitterness and hatred. We must forever conduct our struggle on the high plane of dignity and discipline. We must not allow our creative protest to degenerate into physical violence. Again and again, we must rise to the majestic heights of meeting physical force with soul force.

The marvelous new militancy which has engulfed the Negro community must not lead us to a distrust of all white people, for many of our white brothers, as evidenced by their presence here today, have come to realize that their destiny is tied up with our destiny. And they have come to realize that their freedom is inextricably bound to our freedom.

We cannot walk alone.

And as we walk, we must make the pledge that we shall always march ahead.

We cannot turn back.

There are those who are asking the devotees of civil rights, "When will you be satisfied?" We can never be satisfied as long as the Negro is the victim of the unspeakable horrors of police brutality. We can never be satisfied as long as our bodies, heavy with the fatigue of travel, cannot gain lodging in the motels of the highways and the hotels of the cities. We cannot be satisfied as long as a Negro in Mississippi cannot vote and a Negro in New York believes he has nothing for which to vote. No, no, we are not satisfied, and we will not be satisfied until "justice rolls down like waters, and righteousness like a mighty stream."

I am not unmindful that some of you have come here out of great trials and tribulations. Some of you have come fresh from narrow jail cells. And some of you have come from areas where your quest — quest for freedom left you battered by the storms of persecution and staggered by the winds of police brutality. You have been the veterans of creative suffering. Continue to work with the faith that unearned suffering is redemptive. Go back to Mississippi, go back to Alabama, go back to South Carolina, go back to Georgia, go back to Louisiana, go back to the slums and ghettos of our northern cities, knowing that somehow this situation can and will be changed.

Let us not wallow in the valley of despair, I say to you today, my friends.

And so even though we face the difficulties of today and tomorrow, I still have a dream. It is a dream deeply rooted in the American dream.

I have a dream that one day this nation will rise up and live out the true meaning of its creed: "We hold these truths to be self-evident, that all men are created equal."

I have a dream that one day on the red hills of Georgia, the sons of former slaves and the sons of former slave owners will be able to sit down together at the table of brotherhood.

I have a dream that one day even the state of Mississippi, a state sweltering with the heat of injustice, sweltering with the heat of oppression, will be transformed into an oasis of freedom and justice.

I have a dream that my four little children will one day live in a nation where they will not be judged by the color of their skin but by the content of their character.

I have a dream today!

I have a dream that one day, down in Alabama, with its vicious racists, with its governor having his lips dripping with the words of "interposition" and "nullification" — one day right there in Alabama little black boys and black girls will be able to join hands with little white boys and white girls as sisters and brothers.

I have a dream today!

I have a dream that one day every valley shall be exalted, and every hill and mountain shall be made low, the rough places will be made plain, and the crooked places will be made straight; "and the glory of the Lord shall be revealed and all flesh shall see it together."

This is our hope, and this is the faith that I go back to the South with.

With this faith, we will be able to hew out of the mountain of despair a stone of hope. With this faith, we will be able to transform the jangling discords of our nation into a beautiful symphony of brotherhood. With this faith, we will be able to work together, to pray together, to struggle together, to go to jail together, to stand up for freedom together, knowing that we will be free one day.

And this will be the day—this will be the day when all of God's children will be able to sing with new meaning:

My country 'tis of thee, sweet land of liberty, of thee I sing.

Land where my fathers died, land of the Pilgrim's pride,

From every mountainside, let freedom ring!

And if America is to be a great nation, this must become true.

And so let freedom ring from the prodigious hilltops of New Hampshire.

Let freedom ring from the mighty mountains of New York.

Appendix

Placement: First year
Time: Theory 60 hours

Course Description:

The course I designed to enable students to enhance ability to comprehend spoken and written English (and use English) required for effective communication in their professional work. Students will practice their skills in verbal and written English during clinical and classroom experiences.

Unit	*Time (hours)*	*Learning objectives*	*Content*	*Teaching Learning Activities*	*Assessment methods*
I	10	*Speak and write grammatically correct English	• Review of grammar • Remedial study of grammar • Building vocabulary • Phonetics • Public speaking	*Demonstrate use of dictionary *Classroom conversation *Exercise on use of grammar *Practice in public speaking	-Objective type -Fill in the blanks -Paraphrasing
II	30	*Develop ability to read, understand and express meaningfully, the prescribed text	• Read and comprehend prescribed course books	*Exercise on >Reading >Summarising >Comprehension	-Short answers -Essay types

Contd.

Contd.

III	10	*Develop writing skills	• Various forms of composi- tion # Letter writing # Note taking # Précis writing # Nurses notes # Anecdotal Records # Diary writing # Reports on health problems etc. # Resume/CV	• Exercise on writing • >Letter writing • >Nurses notes • >Précis • >Diary • >Anecdote • >Health problems • >Story writing • >Resume/CV • Essay writing • >Discussion on written reports/ documents	— Assessment of the skills based on the check list
IV	06	* Develop skill in spoken English	• Spoken English >Oral report >Discussion >Debate >Telephonic conversation	* Exercise on > Debating > Participating in seminar, panel, symposium >Telephonic conversation	— Assessment of the skills based on the check list
V	04	*Develop skill in listening compre- hension	• Listening compre- hension media, audio, video, speeches etc.	* Exercise on > Listening to audio, video tapes and identify the key points	— Assessment of the skills based on the check list